THE PARAMEDIC INTERNSHIP GUIDEBOOK

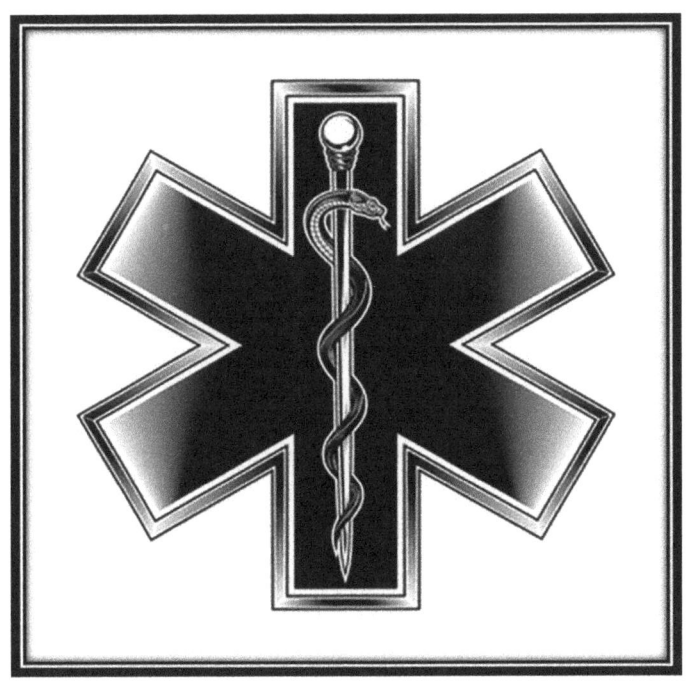

MARK POYER

Copyright © 2022 Mark Poyer
All rights reserved
First Edition

Fulton Books
Meadville, PA

Published by Fulton Books 2022

ISBN 978-1-63985-039-6 (paperback)
ISBN 978-1-63985-040-2 (digital)

Printed in the United States of America

Contents

Page	Topic	Page	Topic	Page	Topic
5	Introduction	62	Trauma	121	Substance Abuse
7	Chest Pain	66	Falls	151	Syncope/Falls
12	Respiratory Distress	69	Motorized Vehicle Accident	156	Allergic Reaction
18	Abdominal Pain	72	Overdose	160	Death in the Field
26	Burns	75	Behavioral	164	Shock
30	Diabetes	78	ETOH	168	Scene Management and MCI
34	Seizures	82	Poisonings	175	Dialysis
40	Stroke/CVA	85	Pain Management	182	ECG Basics
45	Altered Level of Consciousness	93	Pregnancy	186	Home Meds Guide
48	Headache	100	Childbirth	197	EMS Skill Sheets

53	Unresponsiveness	109	Pediatrics	254	Post-Traumatic Stress Disorder
56	Cardiac Arrest	116	Sepsis		

Introduction

Congratulations on getting started on your internship! Going through an internship can be very difficult at times. Not every shift is going to be perfect. Not every call is going to be perfect.

Remember that you are here to learn how to be a paramedic. You are not expected to know how to do that up front. You will, however, be expected to learn and work hard. You will get to a point where you can safely and competently run medical calls. I made this internship guide to be used as a resource to help you become successful in your journey toward becoming a paramedic. This is not specific to any county and can be used as a guide wherever you go. *Remember to follow your county's local protocols and procedures.* I want you to remember that being on an internship is an opportunity. You are working under somebody else's license. I expect you to act professionally and demonstrate that you are here to learn as much as possible. We will work together to make sure you are successful in your endeavor.

How to Use This Book

This book was designed to be used by both the intern and preceptor to help with consistency when it comes to patient assessments and running calls as a student. Think condensed-down paramedic book down to the nitty-gritty. For example, say you're running a chest pain call. Your student missed some questions they should have asked, or maybe they weren't thinking about a certain condition or missed some things regarding differential diagnosis. After the call, you can speak with your student and have them review the short chest pain section. This repetition allows the student to become consistent and gives them clear and concise goals to work toward in becoming a great paramedic.

Understand that this book is not geared toward any one specific county, and it is still recommended that you all follow local protocols, guidelines, and procedures.

Chapter 1

CHEST PAIN

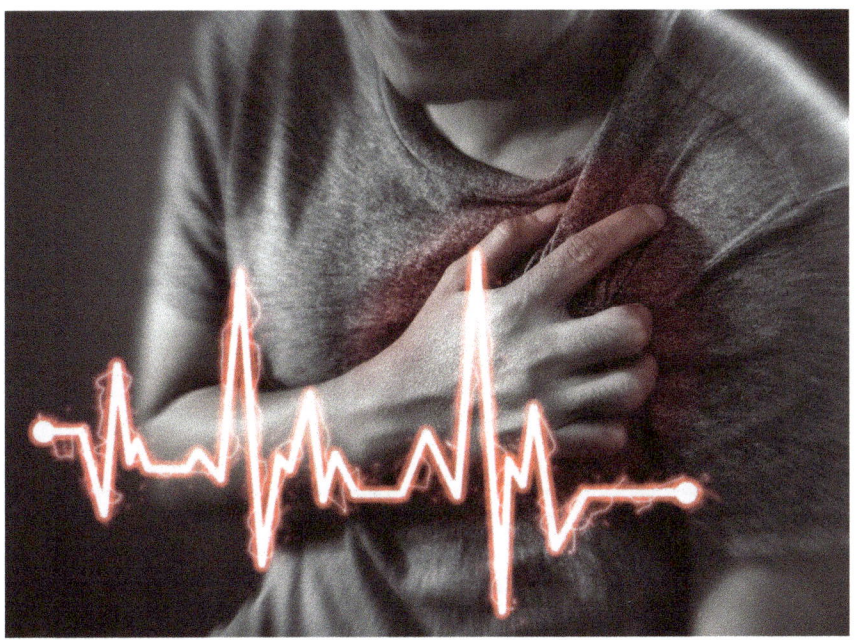

Questions to Ask

1	How long did your chest pain start?
2	What were you doing when your chest pain started?
3	Can you point to where your pain is?
4	Does your pain radiate anywhere else?
5	Can you describe your pain (sharp, pressure, dull aching, stabbing, etc.)?
6	Did the pain come on fast or slowly over time?
7	Does anything make your pain better or worse?
8	How bad is your pain on a scale from 1–10?
9	Are you having any difficulty breathing? If yes, then ask the following questions.
10	Which came on first, the chest pain or the shortness of breath?
11	Does it hurt to take a deep breath? Check lung sounds.
12	Have you had a cough or any sputum production? What color is the sputum?
13	Any fever, body aches, chills, nausea, vomiting, diarrhea, recent illnesses, or trauma?
14	Any cardiac conditions? Pacemaker, heart surgery, arrhythmias, or previous heart attacks?
15	Are you taking any medication? Are you compliant with your medication? Have you recently been prescribed any new medication?

Words of Wisdom

1	Do not let these patients walk. Utilize a stair chair or a gurney.
2	Treat the patient, not the monitor.
3	Always have a backup plan.
4	If you need help, delegate tasks to free yourself up.
5	Patients with ALS complaints receive ALS treatment. Monitor IV, possible drug administration, consider blood sugar, 12-lead ECG, oxygen, or other treatments if appropriate.

Chest Pain Treatment (Follow Local Protocols)

1	Monitor
2	Oxygen (if indicated)
3	Aspirin
4	12-lead ECG and possibly a right-sided ECG
5	Nitroglycerin (if no inferior wall MI, see protocol)
6	IV access
7	Consider morphine or pain management
8	Consider Zofran
9	Consider dopamine for cariogenic shock
10	If positive for MI, transport to a STEMI/STAR center

Differential Diagnosis

Angina	Chest pain that goes away with rest. This usually occurs with stress or physical activity. it is caused by poor blood flow to the heart. Generally caused by blood clots. Angina can be a recurring or acute problem. Typically lasts less than 15 minutes. Unstable angina occurs at rest and can last longer than thirty minutes. People with a history of coronary artery disease (CAD) are prone to have angina because of ischemia to the heart tissue.
Myocardial infarction	Occurs when blood flow to the heart is blocked. When this happens, ischemia occurs, and the heart tissue begins to die. Pain lasts longer than twenty minutes. Very painful, the patient typically feels a heavy pressure like an "elephant sitting on their chest." Pain can radiate to the arms, jaw, and back. Some people such as the elderly, women, and people diagnosed with diabetes may experience little to no chest pain. Look for confirmed ST elevation in two or more leads.
Cardiogenic shock	When the heart is unable to pump efficiently. Most often caused by an MI. Patient's skin signs can be pale, cool, and diaphoretic and should have a low blood pressure systolic below ninety. This is more common in patients with a history of heart failure, diabetes, high blood pressure, and coronary artery disease. Patient may present with crackles in lung fields. Dopamine is typically used for treatment in the field with 5–10 mcg for inotropic doses.

Pericarditis	Inflammation of the pericardium. Patient may need to bend over while breathing. Pain is increased upon respirations. May hear crackles and rubbing sounds when listening to the lungs. Patient may also present with pedal edema and dry cough. Patient may also have a history of either a bacterial or viral infection and may be on antibiotics. Patient may have a fever. Pain typically comes on suddenly and is described as a sharp stabbing pain. Risk factors are increased with MI history.
Cardiac tamponade	Pressure on the heart that occurs when fluid builds up in the space between the heart muscle (myocardium) and the outer covering sac of the heart (pericardium). Can occur due to MI, heart surgery, bacterial or viral pericarditis, dissecting aortic aneurism, or lung cancer. Symptoms are pain upon respiration, shock, hypotension with deep breaths, palpitations, pulsus paradoxus, and distended neck veins. Look for Beck's triad hypertension, muffled heart tones, and distended neck veins.
Sick sinus syndrome	Sinus bradycardia, sinus tachycardia, SVT, sinus pause, or sinus arrest. Symptoms range from chest pain, confusion, dizziness, nausea, vomiting, palpitations, shortness of breath, fatigue, fainting, or syncope.

Chapter 2

RESPIRATORY DISTRESS

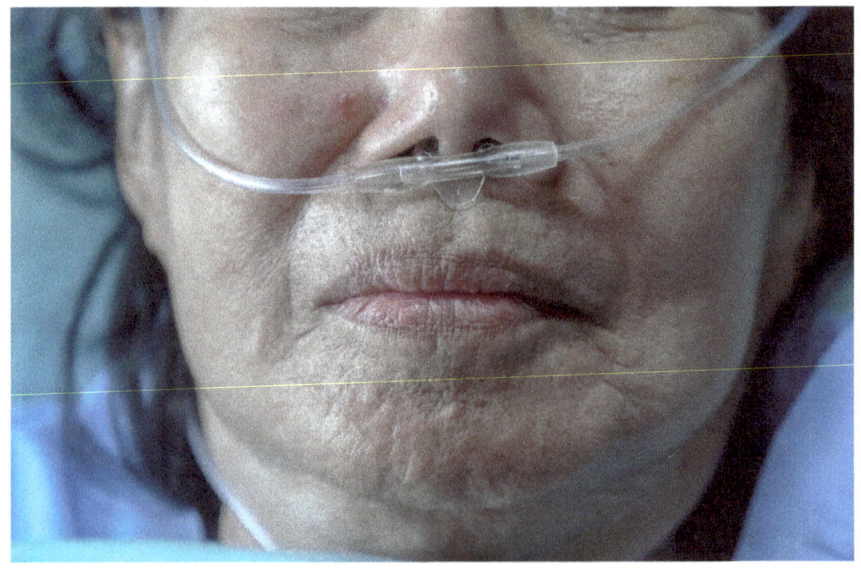

Things to Look for and Think About

1	Remember your ABCs.
2	Respiratory effort: Do they have deep or shallow respirations? Fast or slow respirations? Are they starting to quit?
3	What is the patient's positioning, tripod position, propped up with pillows (COPD), upright, slumped, supine?
4	Any accessory muscle use? Chest, neck, abdomen, or nasal flaring, especially apparent in pediatrics.
5	Do they need oxygen? If so, how will you administer it? Nasal cannula, nonrebreather mask, or BMV on high flow O2?
6	How many words can they speak before having to take another breath?
7	What are their skin signs? Color of nail beds, cyanosis, mottling of the skin, flush, dry, wet, hot, or cold?
8	What is their level of consciousness? Are they alert (hypoxia)?
9	Pay attention to your environment. Do you see any ashtrays or cigarettes lying around, oxygen tanks in the house, or drug paraphernalia? Do you see a CPAP machine? Do you smell smoke?
10	Make sure to get a 12-lead EKG and assess lung sounds. Treat appropriately.
11	Do not let these patients walk. Use a gurney or stair chair so the issue is not exacerbated.

Shortness of Breath Treatment

1	Check ABCs and treat appropriately. Provide oxygen early if appropriate.
2	Assess lung sounds and treat appropriately (Albuterol or CPAP if appropriate).
3	Monitor with spO2 or end tidal taking priority.
4	12-lead ECG.
5	IV, blood sugar, and transport.

Questions to Ask

1	When did the shortness of breath start?
2	What was the patient doing when they became short of breath?
3	Did this come on quickly, or have they been progressively becoming more short of breath over a long period of time?
4	Any chest pain? Does the pain increase when they breathe?
5	Do they get short of breath upon exertion?
6	Has the patient ever been intubated before?
7	Any recent illnesses?
8	Do they have a productive cough with sputum production? If so, what color is the sputum? Any blood?
9	Any fever, body aches, or chills?

10	Any cardiac history or history of any respiratory issues?
11	Any recent trauma?
12	Are they taking any medications? Are they compliant with their medications?

Differential Diagnosis

Congestive heart failure	<ul><li>Increased shortness of breath with everyday tasks</li><li>Waking up in the middle of the night with shortness of breath</li><li>Sleeping propped up with pillows</li><li>Shortness of breath becomes worse with supine position</li><li>Pedal edema</li></ul>
Chronic obstructive pulmonary disease	Bronchitis—blue bloater, inflammation of the bronchial tubes which produces a lot of mucus. Patient typically has a productive cough with sputum production and a hard time getting air in and out of the lungs. Patient can become cyanotic.
Emphysema	Pink puffer—gradually damages the air sacs (alveoli) in your lungs, making it progressively more difficult to breathe. Inner wall sacs weaken and rupture, thus, reducing the amount of oxygen reaching the bloodstream. Smoking is the leading cause of emphysema. Patient is constantly short of breath even while at rest and is typically on oxygen.

Pneumothorax	Typically due to trauma or can be spontaneous because of blebs on the lungs. Typically happens in tall males. There is unequal rise and fall of the chest, decreased or absent lung sounds, unequal pulses, low blood pressure, sudden onset, or worsening. Patient needs needle decompression between the second and third intercostal muscle midclavicular or between the fourth and fifth intercostal space midaxillary. Pneumothorax can occur from trauma such as broken ribs, look for flail chest segment; blunt force trauma, and can occur from flying or diving.
Pulmonary embolism	<ul><li>When one or more of the pulmonary arteries in your lungs becomes blocked.</li><li>Normally caused by blood clots that travel from the legs to the lungs</li><li>Almost always occurs in conjunction with deep vein thrombosis (DVT)</li><li>Signs and symptoms are shortness of breath and chest pain that is worse upon respiration (pleurisy)</li><li>Pain gets worse upon exertion and will not go away with rest.</li><li>Productive cough with blood-tinged sputum</li><li>Common in patients with long periods of immobility, recent surgeries, atrial fibrillation, smoking, and overweight.</li></ul>

Pneumonia	Lung infection caused by bacteria, viruses, or fungi. Common symptoms include greenish, yellowish, or blood-tinged sputum with a productive cough (put a mask on these patients), fever which can be high, body aches, chills, shortness of breath, sharp chest pain, and pale and clammy skin signs. Typically controlled by bed rest and NSAIDS.

Continuous positive airway pressure (CPAP) maintains a continuous level of positive airway pressure in a spontaneously breathing patient. Functionally like PEEP except PEEP is applied pressure against exhalation and CPAP is a constant flow. It is used with people who have breathing problems such as sleep apnea. It is also used for CHF, asthma, COPD, drownings, and pulmonary infections. Know your CPAP procedure in your own county indications, contraindications, etc.

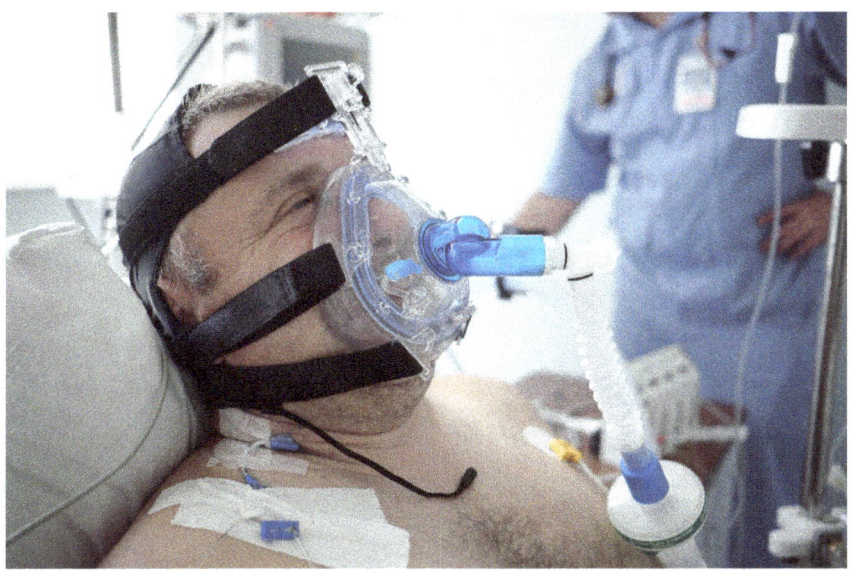

Chapter 3

ABDOMINAL PAIN

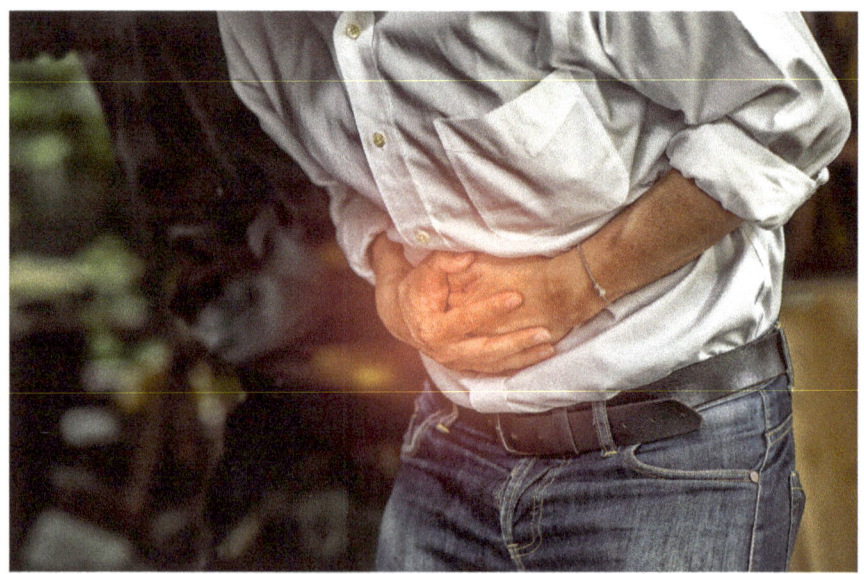

Questions to Ask

1	When did the pain start?
2	What were you doing when the pain started?
3	Does anything make it better or worse?
4	Can you describe the pain?
5	Can you point to where the pain is?
6	Does the pain radiate or go anywhere else?
7	How bad is your pain on a scale from 1–10?
8	Any nausea, vomiting, diarrhea, or painful urination? If painful urination, ask about any history of UTIs or a recent fever. Assess for possible sepsis.
9	Have you been able to eat or hold fluids down? When was the last time you ate or had something to drink?
10	Any possibility of food poisoning?
11	Any history of being diabetic? If so, check their sugar and ask them when the last time they checked their sugar was.
12	Has this pain ever happened to them before? Did they go to the hospital? What did the hospital say?
13	If the patient is a female, is there any chance of pregnancy? Do they take any birth control medication?
14	When was their last menstrual period?
15	Any abnormal vaginal bleeding or discharge?
16	Any recent illnesses or trauma?

Bowel Questions

1	When was your last bowel movement?
2	Any changes in frequency?
3	Solid or loose stools?
4	Unusual odor or color? Any blood in the stool?

Bladder Questions

1	When did you urinate last?
2	Any changes in frequency?
3	Does it hurt to pee? Any burning sensation?
4	Any discoloration or unusual odors? Any blood in the urine?
5	Is it difficult to start or stop urinating?
6	Do you have a history of urinary tract infections or kidney stones?
7	Any fever, body aches, or chills?
8	If so, are they currently taking any antibiotics?

Abdominal Pain Treatment

1	Consider ABCs
2	Focused assessment

3	Monitor
4	Vital signs
5	IV if appropriate
6	Normal saline if hypotensive, or dehydrated, or hyperglycemic
7	Zofran if appropriate
8	Pain medication if appropriate

Differential Diagnosis

Appendicitis	Inflammation of the appendix. Pain occurs in the lower right quadrant and typically radiates to the navel. McBurney's point is the point between the anterior and superior iliac spine to the navel and is the location of the pain with appendicitis. Most often occurs in patients between the ages of ten to thirty. Treatment is the surgical removal of the appendix. Pain typically worsens with movement and coughing. Expect nausea or vomiting, low-grade fever, constipation or diarrhea, and abdominal bloating. In pregnant women, the appendix is higher and may seem like the pain is in the upper right quadrant. Pain is severe. If not removed quickly, the appendix can rupture from all the bacteria and will cause inflammation.
Upper GI bleed	Coffee ground emesis—bleeding arising from the esophagus, stomach, or duodenum—can be caused by peptic ulcers, gastric erosion, esophageal varices, and gastric cancer.

Lower GI bleed	Involves the colon and small intestine. Bleeding from the last first or fourth of the duodenum, jejunum, ileum, colon, and rectum. Expect black tar-like stools known as melena or bright red stools (hematochezia). Patient can be in shock, have an altered mental status, MI, weakness, and fainting or syncope.
Ectopic pregnancy	When a fertilized egg is implanted outside of the uterus. This is life-threatening. Lots of blood loss can occur. Abdominal pain, pelvic pain, and light vaginal bleeding are often the first warning signs of an ectopic pregnancy. Extreme dizziness and fainting can occur. Ectopic pregnancies typically occur in the first eight to ten weeks of pregnancy. Patient needs an ultrasound and surgery to remove the fallopian tube if it is a tubular pregnancy. This is treated with laparoscopic surgery. If the tube is not significantly damaged, it can be repaired after the extraction of the fetus.
Ulcers	Painful sores in the lining of the stomach or the first part of the stomach called the duodenum. Can be caused by an infection and use of NSAIDS. Can cause burning pain in the middle or upper stomach, bloating, heartburn, nausea, or vomiting. Severe cases can have severe abdominal pain or melena. Patients will normally get an acid-blocking medication used for heartburn. Patient may need an upper endoscopy (looking through the throat into the stomach to look for abnormalities). Treated with lifestyle changes, limiting dairy, medication, or surgery. Patient may be on proton pump inhibitors or antibiotics.

Abdominal aortic aneurysm	The aorta is the body's main supplier of blood. If ruptured, it will cause life-threatening bleeding within seconds. The aneurysm grows slowly and without symptoms. When enlarged, a pulsating feeling near the navel may be felt. Patients will normally have a deep constant pain in their abdomen with back pain. You may also see a narrowing pulse pressure or a pulsating mass. Check for equal pulses in the patient's extremities. Smoking significantly increases your risk of having AAA. Causing factors include tobacco use, hardening of the arteries (atherosclerosis), or infection of the aorta (vasculitis). AAAs most often occur in people over the age of sixty-five; more common in males. Expect sudden intense abdominal pain if the aorta bursts, expect shock, ALOC, and shortness of breath. Patient needs chest X-ray, ultrasound, MRI, and open abdominal surgery.
Cholecystitis	• Inflammation of the gallbladder • Fair, fat, and forty females eating fatty meals • Can be life-threatening • Treatment is often the removal of the gallbladder • Symptoms: RUQ pain, pain radiates to the right shoulder or back • Tenderness over the abdomen when palpated • Nausea or vomiting and fever • Caused by gallstones (hard particles that develop in your gallbladder) • Blocks cystic ducts which bile flows out of • Bile begins to build up, resulting in inflammation

	• Can be caused by a tumor, bile duct blockage • Treatment for gallstones is often antibiotics, fasting, surgery to remove gallbladder, or a laparoscopic cholecystectomy
Kidney stones	Small hard deposits that form inside of your kidneys. Kidney stones can affect any part of your urinary tract. Treatment is typically pain medication and fluids. Symptoms are severe abdominal or back pain; pain comes in waves; pain upon urination; pink, red, or brown urine; urinating more than usual; nausea or vomiting; or difficulty passing urine. Types of kidney stones—calcium stones, strive stones, uric acid stones, and cystine stones. Risk factors—common in males ages forty and up. Caused by diet that is high in protein, sodium, sugar, and obesity. Sound waves can be used to break up the kidney stones. Surgical removal of the stones is possible.
Ovarian cysts	Fluid-filled sacs or pockets within or on the surface of an ovary. Symptoms include pelvic pain, pain during intercourse, pain during bowel movements, nausea or vomiting, pressure on the bladder, and frequent urination. Treatment may require surgery, birth control pills, and waiting. Cysts typically go away on their own after a couple of months.
Pelvic inflammatory disease	An infection of female reproductive organs. Usually occurs when sexually transmitted bacteria spread from the vagina to the uterus, fallopian tubes, or ovaries. Symptoms—pain in lower abdomen and pelvis, heavy vaginal discharge, irregular menstrual bleeding, pain

	during intercourse, fever, and difficulty urinating. Most often caused by gonorrhea or chlamydia infections. Risk factors—sexually active, multiple sex partners, and incorrectly inserted IUD. Patient needs ultrasound. Treatment is normally antibiotics.
Hernia	Occurs when an organ or fatty tissue squeezes through a weak spot in a surrounding muscle or connective tissue called fascia. Symptoms—abnormal vaginal discharge, painful intercourse, painful urination, foul odor, back pain, and fever. Bulge with a burning or aching sensation. Normally occurs in the groin.

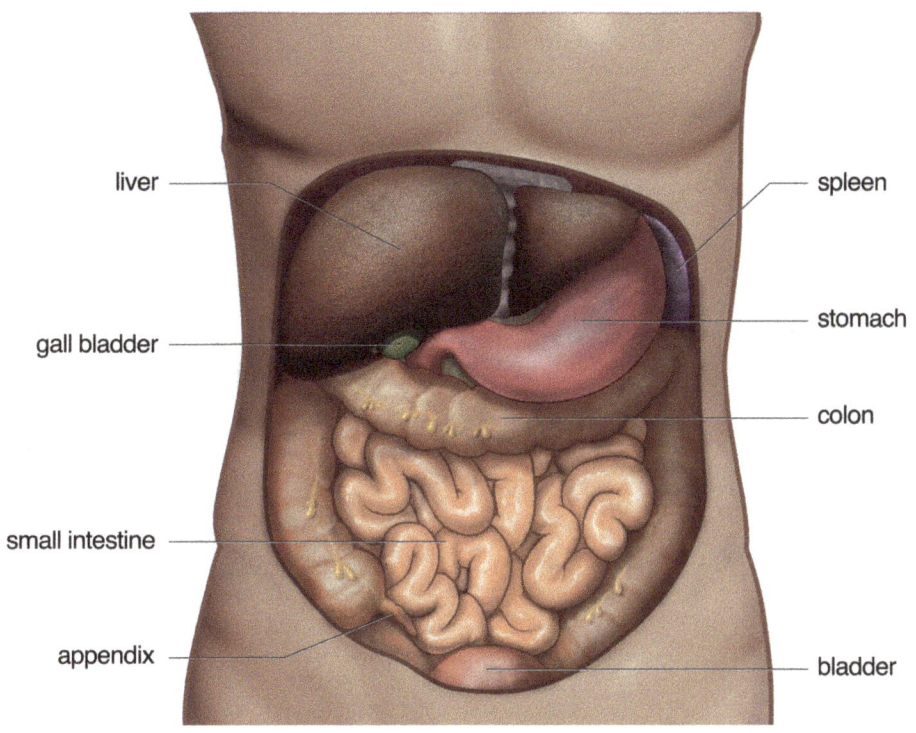

Chapter 4

BURNS

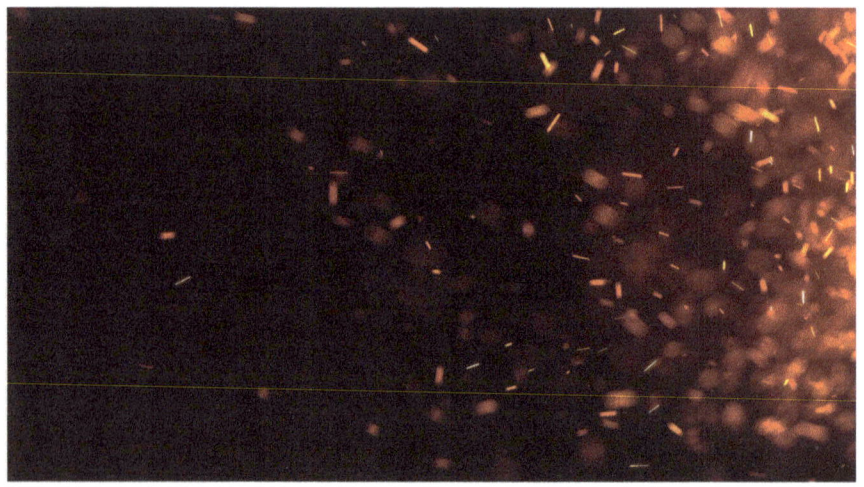

Rule of Nines

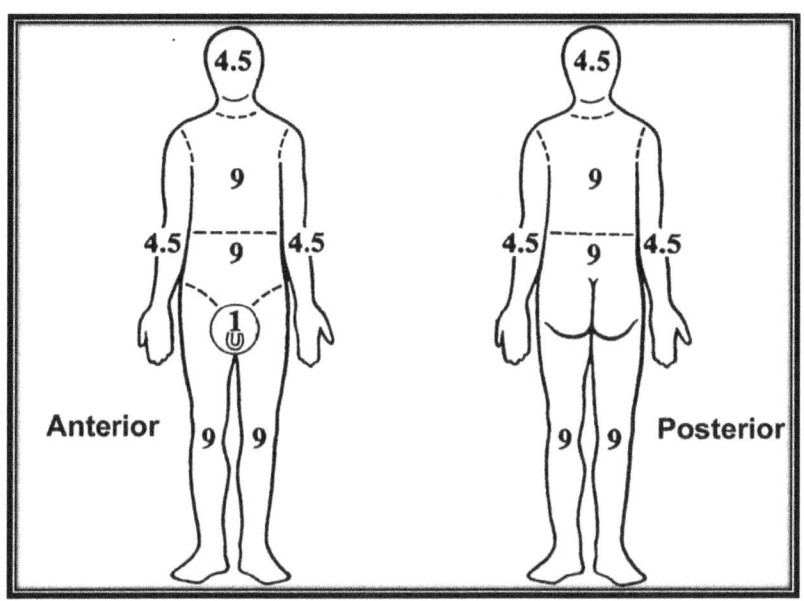

Patient's Palm = 1% TBSA

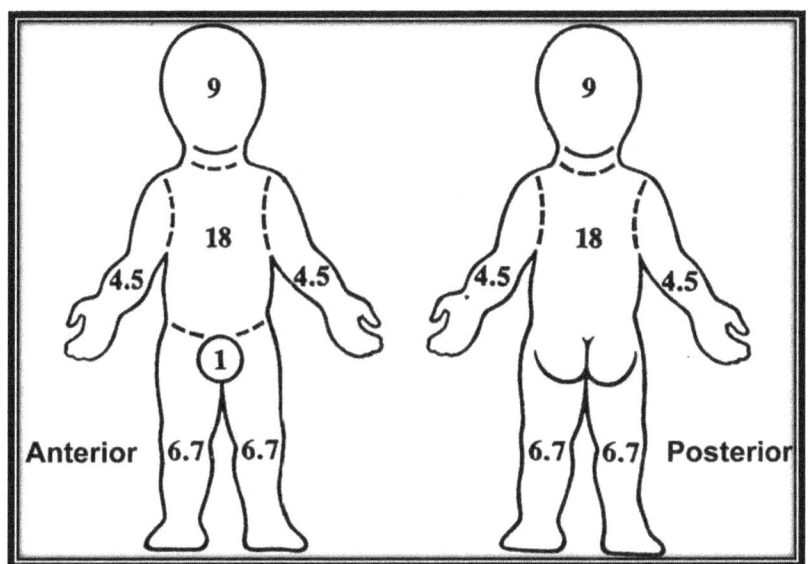

What to Look For

1	ABCs
2	Level of consciousness
3	Respiratory involvement, singed nostrils, burned airway, smoke inhalation, black sputum, hoarseness
4	Location and percentage of burns (patient palm = 1% TBSA
5	Any trauma
6	Laryngeal edema
7	Full vs. partial
8	Entrance or exit wound if electrical

Info to Get

1	Symptoms
2	What kind of burn is it, thermal, chemical, electrical, or steam?
3	When, where, and how did it happen?
4	Was it in an enclosed space? How long were they exposed to the smoke if any?
5	Estimated patient weight

Burn Information

First-degree burn	Skin is usually red (superficial burn), often there is swelling, and pain is sometimes present.
Second-degree burn	Burn through the first and second layers of skin (dermis). Blisters develop, skin is reddened and splotchy in appearance, severe pain, and swelling.
Third-degree burn	Most serious burns that involve all layer of the skin—fat, muscle, and bone may be affected. Areas may be charred black or appear dry and white.

Burn Fluid Formulas

Parkland formula	TBSA burned % × weight in kg × 4 ml. Give ½ of total fluid requirements in the first eight hours and the rest over the next sixteen hours.
Alfred prehospital fluid formula	Total amount in ml = weight in kg × TBSA %

Chapter 5

DIABETES

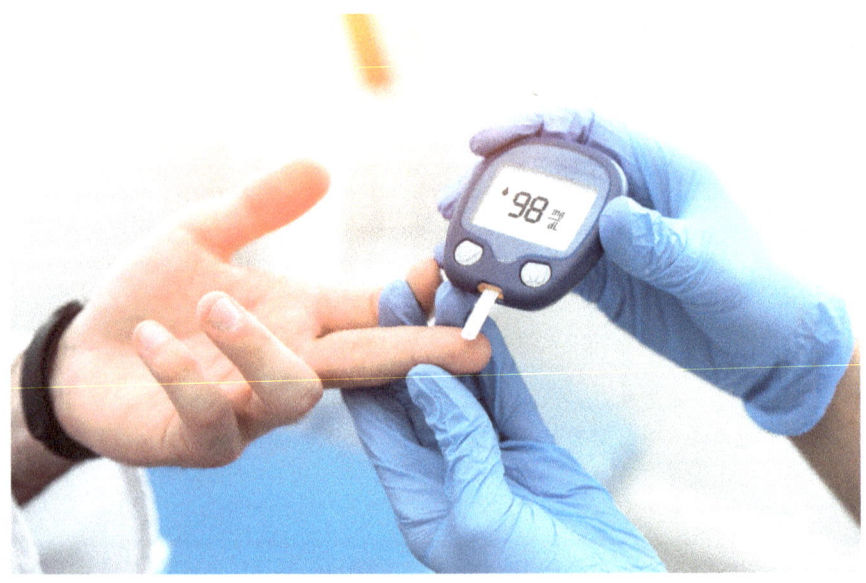

What to Look For

1	The three Ps—polyphagia, polydipsia, polyuria > DKA indication
2	Fruity odor
3	Skin signs
4	Altered level of consciousness
5	Respiratory effort

Questions to Ask

1	What is going on today?
2	When did the symptoms start?
3	History of diabetes?
4	Are they on diabetic medication?
5	Are they type 1 or type 2?
6	If they are insulin dependent, when was their last dose?
7	How much insulin did they get?
8	When was their last meal?
9	Have they noticed an increase or decrease in appetite or thirst?
10	When did the patient last check their blood sugar?

Type 1 diabetes	Usually diagnosed in children and young adults. Body does not produce insulin. The body's immune system attacks and destroys the pancreas's insulin-producing cells. Lifelong insulin injections are required to control blood sugar.
Type 2 diabetes	The pancreas loses the ability to appropriately produce and release insulin. The body also becomes resistant to insulin, and the blood sugar rises. Most common form of diabetes.
Pancreas	A gland organ. It is part of the digestion system and produces important enzymes and hormones that help break down foods. The pancreas also produces insulin and secretes it into the bloodstream.
Hyperglycemia	1. High blood sugar typically reads Hi when above five hundred on a glucometer. 2. Three Ps—polyphagia, polydipsia, polyuria. 3. Failure to treat diabetic ketoacidosis will result in a diabetic coma. 4. Ketoacidosis occurs when your body does not have enough insulin. Without insulin, your body cannot use glucose as fuel, so your body breaks down fats to use for energy. When fat breaks down, ketones are produced. Your body cannot tolerate large amounts of ketones and will try and eliminate it through the urine. When there are too many ketones and cannot be released, it leads to DKA.

Hypoglycemia	1) Glucose level below sixty. 2) Also referred to as an insulin reaction or insulin shock. 3) Hypoglycemia can lead to coma or death (treat as early as possible). 4) Signs and symptoms—ALOC, sweating or chills, anxiety, irritability, tachycardia, dizziness, hunger, headache, blurred vision, weakness, fatigue, ataxia, seizures, tingling, numbness in lips or tongue. 5) Patient may appear intoxicated.
Diabetic medications	• Increase insulin production—Diabinese, Glucotrol, Micromase, Diabeta, Glynase, Amaryl, Prandin, and Starlix • Decrease insulin production—Glucophage and Avandia • Injectable—Novalog and Novalin

Diabetes Type 2 Medication Classes

Class	Common Drugs	Mechanism	Hypoglycemia
Biguanides	Metformin	Decreases hepatic gluconeogenesis	No
Sulfonylureas	Glyburide, Glipizide	Increases insulin secretion	Yes
Thiazolidinediones	Pioglitazone, Rosiglitazone	Increases insulin sensitivity in muscle and fat	No
Meglitinides	Repaglinide, Nateglinide	Increases insulin secretion	Yes
α-glucosidase inhibitors	Acarbose, Miglitol	Decreases intestinal absorption of carbohydrates	No
DPP-4 inhibitors	Sitagliptin, Saxagliptin	Increases insulin secretion	Yes
Incretin mimetics	Exenatide	Increases insulin secretion	Yes
Insulin	Regular, Lispro, Aspart, NPH, Glargine	Increases glucose uptake	Yes

Chapter 6

SEIZURES

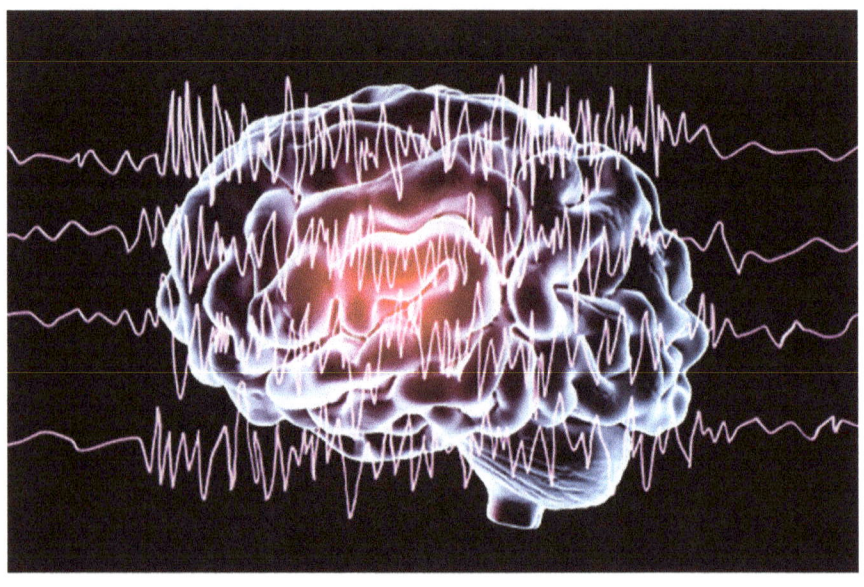

Things to Look For

1	Possible trauma
2	Bystanders that witnessed the incident
3	Incontinence
4	Oral trauma
5	Postictal state
6	Medical alert jewelry

Questions to Ask

1	Ask bystanders if any what they witnessed.
2	How long did the seizure last?
3	Were there multiple seizures?
4	Was it a grand mal seizure? Was their whole body shaking?
5	Did the patient fall and hit their head? Look for trauma. Consider C-spine protocol.
6	Were they complaining of anything prior to the seizure happening?
7	Did they stop breathing at any point? (Consider oxygen if long-lasting seizure.)
8	Does the patient have a history of seizures (alcohol related, epilepsy, or othemeurological disorder)?
9	Have they prescribed any medication for their seizures? Are they compliant?
10	What medication are they taking? Any recent changes to their dosage?
11	When was their last seizure?
12	Has anything changed with the seizures? Activity, length of seizure, frequency?

Seizure Differential Diagnosis

1	Cardiac arrhythmias
2	Hyperglycemia/hypoglycemia
3	Drug/alcohol withdrawal
4	Toxic ingestion/substance abuse
5	Meningitis/encephalitis
6	Head injury
7	Hyperthermia/hypothermia
8	Hypoxia

Aura	Happens before the seizure; may alert the person of an oncoming seizure. Typically begins seconds before the seizure occurs. Some auras are unusual feelings, abnormal sensations, forced thinking, perceived sounds, tastes, or smells. Physical sensations can be dizziness, headache, numbness, light-headedness, and nausea.
Ictus	The convulsive state commonly known as the grand mal stage or a nonconvulsive seizure such as staring or inability to respond normally.
Postictal	Occurs after the ictus stage of the seizure. During this stage, the body begins to relax, and aftereffects may set in. After effects may include numbness, headache, fatigue, drowsiness, partial paralysis, confusion, agitation, loss of consciousness, unresponsiveness, or incontinence.

Stages of a Seizure

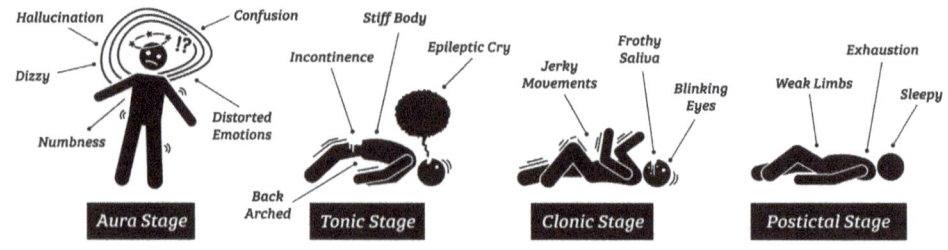

Types of Seizures

Tonic-clonic seizures	Aka grand mal seizure. This involves a loss of consciousness, stiffening of the body, shaking, and jerking movements, sometimes followed by incontinence.
Tonic seizure	Includes body stiffening but does not include the clonic phase of uncontrolled jerking or spasms. Back, arms, and leg muscles are most often affected. Seizure may cause the patient to fall or collapse.
Clonic seizure	Includes jerking muscle movements that are more rhythmic than chaotic. The muscle spasms typically affect the face, neck, and arms and may last for several minutes.
Myoclonic seizure	Typically short and involve uncontrollable jerking usually of the arms and legs and only lasts for a second or two.
Absence seizure	Aka petit mal seizures. The patient may seem to disconnect from the world and blank out for a few seconds. People usually lose

	awareness for a short time and have no memory of the seizure afterward.
Atonic seizure	Aka drop attacks, drop seizures, or kinetic epileptic drop attacks. May involve sudden loss of muscle tone, head drop, or leg weakening. May cause a patient to collapse or drop objects.
Simple partial seizure	Aka simple focal seizure. May only include the aura. During this type of seizure, awareness, memory, or consciousness remains intact. It may result in involuntary jerking of a body part or tingling and may include dizziness.
Complex partial seizure	Aka psychomotor seizure. They alter consciousness or responsiveness. The person having the seizure may appear to be staring into space or moving without a purpose. Some common movements include hand rubbing, chewing, swallowing, and repetitive movements such as walking in a circle.
Status epilepticus	Seizure lasting more than five minutes or several seizures back-to-back without regaining consciousness.

Seizure Treatment

1	Oxygen if appropriate
2	Monitor
3	Blood sugar
4	IV
5	Anticonvulsant such as midazolam if appropriate

Chapter 7

STROKE/CVA

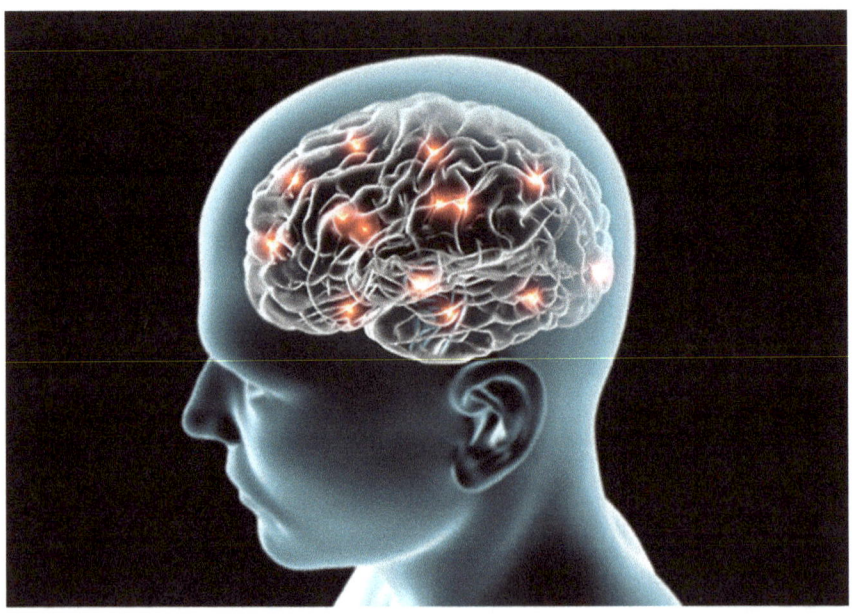

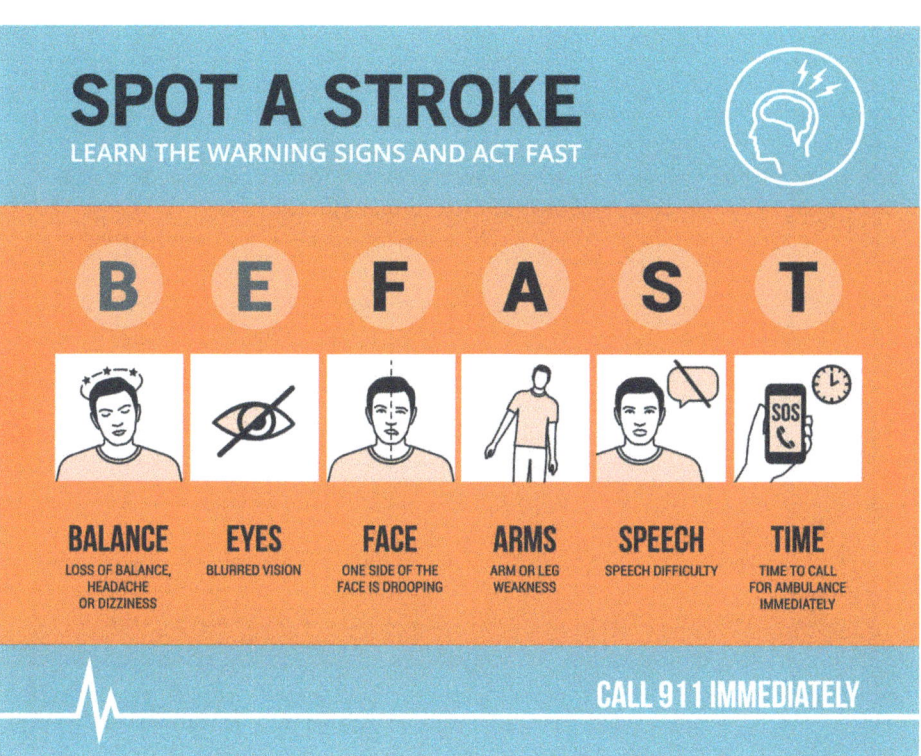

Acronym: What to Look For

B	Blood glucose
E	Eyes (diplopia), blurred vision
F	Facial droop
A	Arm drift
S	Speech abnormalities or slurred speech
T	Time last seen normal or time of onset

Questions to Ask

1	When was the patient last seen normal?
2	Has the patient ever had a stroke before?
3	Any deficiencies from the previous stroke?
4	Any complaints of headache, dizziness, weakness, blurred vision, or nausea/vomiting?
5	What were they doing when it first started?
6	Did the patient fall? Head-to-toe assessment to rule out trauma for possible head injury.
7	Consider C-spine precautions
8	If witnessed by bystanders, was there any shaking on the ground? Rule out seizures.
9	What medications are they taking? Are they compliant? Any new medications? Any substance or drug abuse?
10	Any blood thinners? Any recent surgeries?
11	Any chest pain or shortness of breath?

Types of Strokes Information

Ischemic stroke	Occurs because of an obstruction within a blood vessel supplying blood to the brain. The underlying condition for this obstruction is the development of fatty deposits lining the vessel walls. Aka atherosclerosis.

These fatty deposits cause two types of obstruction:

1. Cerebral thrombosis—which refers to a thrombus (blood clot) that develops at the clogged part of the vessel.
2. Cerebral embolism—refers to a blood clot that forms at another location in the circulatory system. Usually occurs in the heart and large arteries; sometimes caused by atrial fibrillation.

Types of Strokes Information

Hemorrhagic stroke	Results from a weakened blood vessel that ruptures and bleeds into the surrounding brain. The blood accumulates and compresses the surrounding brain tissue. Two types of hemorrhage strokes: 1. Intracerebral hemorrhage (within the brain tissue) 2. Subarachnoid hemorrhage Hemorrhagic stroke can occur from an aneurysm, which is the ballooning of a weakened region of a blood vessel, and if left untreated, it will continue to weaken until it ruptures and bleeds into the brain.

Types of Strokes Information

Transient ischemic stroke	Aka a ministroke that is caused by a clot; however, the clot is transient (temporary). Symptoms occur rapidly and last for a shorttime. Most TIAs last less than five minutes, average being about a minute. Normally does not result in permanent damage.

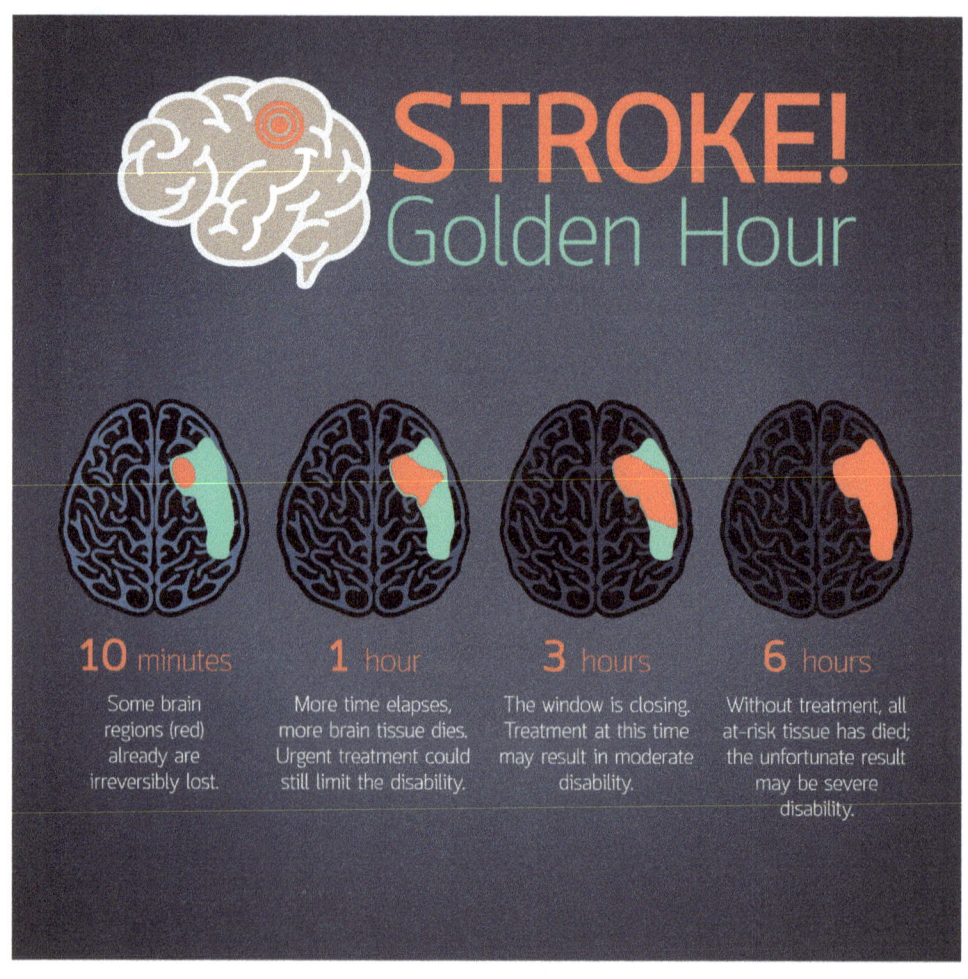

Chapter 8

ALTERED LEVEL OF CONSCIOUSNESS

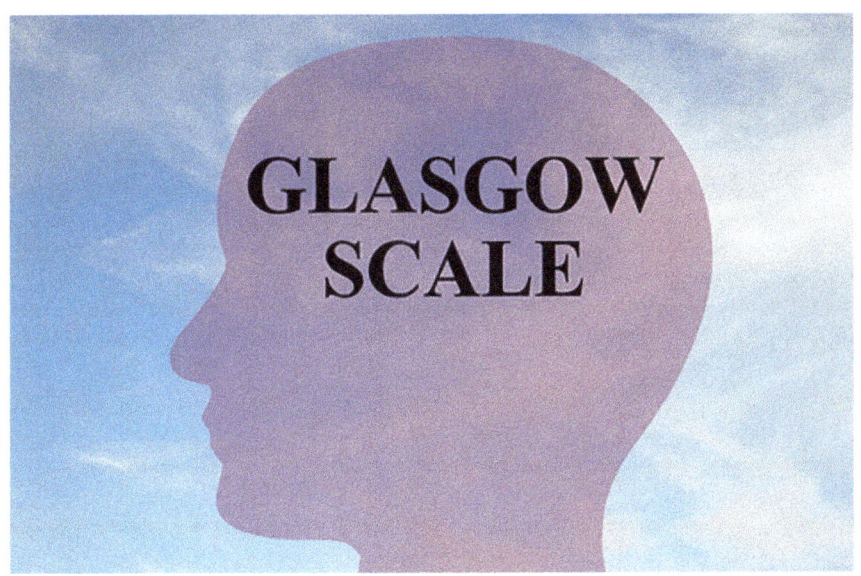

What to Look for and What to Think About

1	Signs of any trauma and a possible mechanism of injury
2	Pupil or breathing abnormalities
3	Track marks, drug paraphernalia
4	Empty bottles—alcohol, pills, or anything the patient can ingest
5	Incontinence
6	Medical alert tags
7	Oral trauma (possibility of a seizure)
8	Any bystanders that witness anything?
9	Does the bystander know anything about the patient? Normal mental status?
10	If so when was the patient last seen normal?
11	What are their A&O status and their GCS score?
12	Is the patient a diabetic? Check blood sugar.

Differential Diagnosis: Altered Level of Consciousness

A	Alcohol	Smell of ETOH, bottles lying around
E	Epilepsy	Eye twitching, ALOC, oral trauma, incontinence
I	Insulin	ABGL (abnormal blood glucose levels), hyper/hypoglycemia

O	Overdose	a) Opioid—pinpoint pupils, decreased respiratory rate, track marks b) TCA—hot as hell, dry as a bone, red as a beet, mad as a hatter c) Benzodiazepine—CNS depressant, double vision, coma, respiratory depression, bradycardia, hypotension, hypothermia d) Cocaine—increased blood pressure, paranoia, MI, coma, stroke, increased heart rate, seizure (See drug section for more info.)
U	Underdose	Empty pill bottles, not compliant with medications
T	Trauma	MOI, head injury, ALOC, signs of bleeding, hypoperfusion
I	Infection	Sepsis, fever, body aches, chills, nausea/vomiting, lethargy
P	Psychosis/poisoning	Abnormal pupils, abnormal heart rate, and abnormal respiratory rate, ALOC, sludge symptoms, abdominal pain
S	Stroke/seizure	Postictal state, complaints of headache, unequal pupils, abnormal stroke scale

Chapter 9

HEADACHE

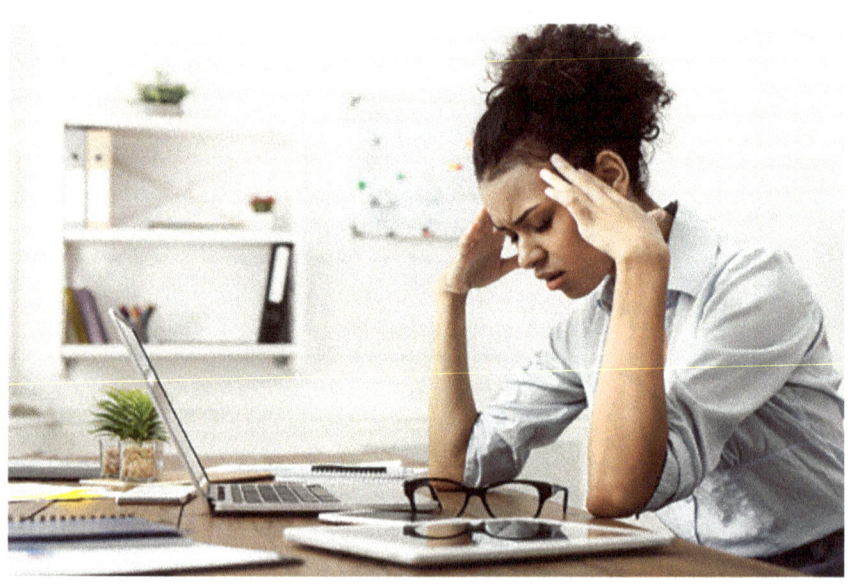

Differential Diagnosis

Cluster headaches	The most painful kind of headache. The pain is severe, quality, and typically located behind the eyes or on the temples. Patients have described it as being sorely painful than childbirth. Patients have also described it as having a red-hot poker inserted into the eye or a spike penetrating down from the top of the head. Causes can be from the following: 1. *Vascular*—pain from dilation of blood vessels which creates pressure on the trigeminal nerve 2. *Hypothalamus*—due to an abnormality in the hypothalamus that is responsive to light/day, smell, steroids, corticosteroids, and neurotransmitted information arising from the heart, stomach, reproductive system, or stress 3. *Genetic*—first-degree relatives are more likely to have the condition. 4. *Triggers*—alcohol, MSG, smells, sleep, diet, NTG 5. *Smoking*—heavy addiction to smoking
Tension headache	The most common headaches are normally caused by tight, contracted muscles in your shoulders, neck, scalp, and jaw. They are often related to stress, depression, anxiety, overworking, not getting enough sleep, missing meals, or using alcohol or drugs.

Migraine	There are four phases of a migraine that are listed below that are common. Not all patients will experience all these symptoms: 1. *The prodrome*—which occurs hours or days before the headache begins. These patients typically experience an altered mood, depression, sleepiness, fatigue, yawning, or stiff muscles in the neck. 2. *The aura*—which immediately precedes the headache (visual/auditory disturbances, pins and needles feeling, hypersensitive to touch, vertigo). 3. *The pain phase*—nausea, light sensitivity, blurred vision, delirium, diarrhea, frequent urination, pale skin, or sweating. 4. *The postdrome*—patient may feel tired or hungover, cognitive difficulties, GI symptoms, mood changes, or weakness.
Hypoxia	Cerebral hypoxemia, especially when coupled with an increase in carbon dioxide tension in the blood, results in extreme dilation of cerebral vessels, notably of the arteries and the arterioles.
Sinus Headache	Sinus headaches can cause pain in the front of your head and face. They are due to inflammation of the sinus passages that lie behind the cheeks, nose, and eyes. The pain tends to be worse when you bend forward or just wake up in the morning. Postnasal drip, sore throat, and nasal discharge typically occur with these headaches.

Blood Sugar	When blood sugar levels are not consistent and have extreme ups and downs, a headache can be triggered. This intense fluctuation both increases and decreases insulin levels, leading to problems with the regulation of other hormones known as epinephrine and norepinephrine. Blood vessels in your brain begin to expand and contract, and a headache occurs.
Stroke	Can be caused by ischemia to the brain or inflammation caused by hemorrhage causing brain tissues to swell. May also be hypertensive.
Dehydration	The human brain is more than 75 percent water and is very sensitive to the amount of water available to it. When the brain detects that the water supply is too low, it begins to produce histamines. This is essentially a process of water rationing and conservation to safeguard the brain in case water shortage continues for a long period of time. The histamines directly cause pain and fatigue.
Medication	Reaction to medication from blood vessels dilating, fluctuation in hormones, and hydration.
Cardiac/hypercapnia	Excess CO_2 will cause relaxation of cerebrovascular smooth muscle and lead to vasodilation and increased ICP.
Alcohol	Ethanol (the type of alcohol in beer, wine, and other alcohol) has an immediate effect on the blood vessels in the body. It causes the vessels to dilate, leading to the flushing feeling many drinkers get with their first drink. Dilation of the blood vessels in the brain may cause headaches, and alcohol is considered to be a trigger for migraines.

Diet	Allergies to foods and imbalance of micro-nutrients in the body such as nutrients and vitamins.
Infection	Any eye, ear, or sinus infection can put pressure around the face and head, resulting in muscle aches and pains and leads to headaches. Encephalitis and meningitis are viruses that affect the brain, and both may cause severe headaches. The membrane surrounding the brain usually becomes extremely inflamed, and prompt medical attention is imperative. Any inflammation that occurs in the brain can put intense pressure on the nerves.
Electrolytes	The more common ions needed for the human body are sodium bicarbonate or chloride, magnesium, potassium, and calcium. They are required by the cells to regulate the electric charge and flow of the water molecules across the cell membrane. Imbalances of electrolytes can cause headaches.

Chapter 10

UNRESPONSIVENESS

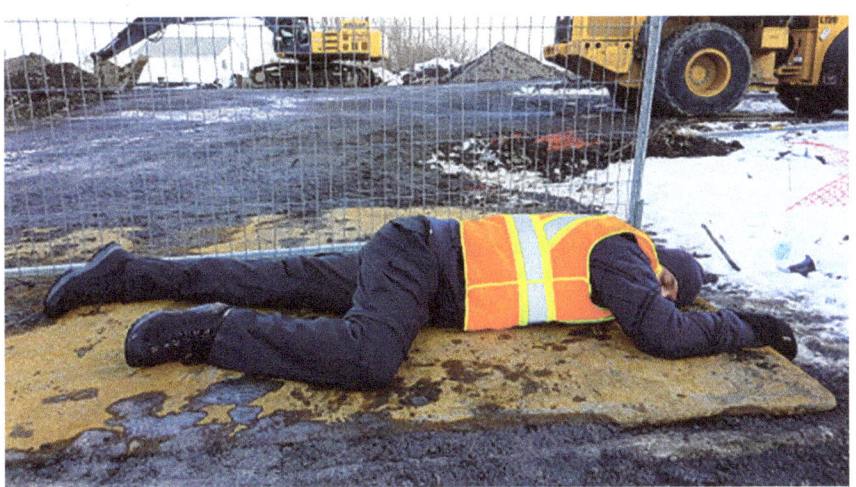

Questions to Ask

1	*Make sure to assess ABCs* and find out how long they have been down.
2	Were there any complaints prior to them becoming unresponsive?
3	What were they doing prior to becoming unresponsive?
4	Were they standing, sitting, or lying down prior?
5	Did anyone see them fall? Did they lose consciousness prior to the fall or after? (Check for trauma/C spine)
6	Did anyone notice any shaking or seizure-like activity?
7	Any recent trauma or illnesses?
8	What kind of medical history do they have? Utilize bystanders who may know.
9	What medications are they taking? Are they compliant? Any substance or drug abuse?
10	*Check pupils*

Differential Diagnosis and Treatments

Respiratory or cardiac arrest	Treat appropriately
Hypoglycemia	Monitor blood sugar, IV, dextrose, or possibly glucagon
Hypovolemia	Monitor large-bore IV wide open with NS and BP before and after

Seizures	Midazolam IV or IM if active and monitor. Follow seizure protocol.
Trauma	Rapid trauma assessment, IV, titrate pressure to 90 systolic, and treat other findings appropriately such as bleeding control or tension pneumothorax
Overdose	Follow protocol, .4–2 mg of Narcan IV, IM, or IN. May repeat. Zofran for nausea if indicated. TCA overdose 1 MEQ/kg IV/IO. Follow local protocols.
CVA/stroke	Stroke screen, monitor (expect to see hypertension and a CC of a headache), IV, and 12-lead transport code 3 if within time window
ETOH	Monitor and treat signs and symptoms.

Chapter 11

CARDIAC ARREST

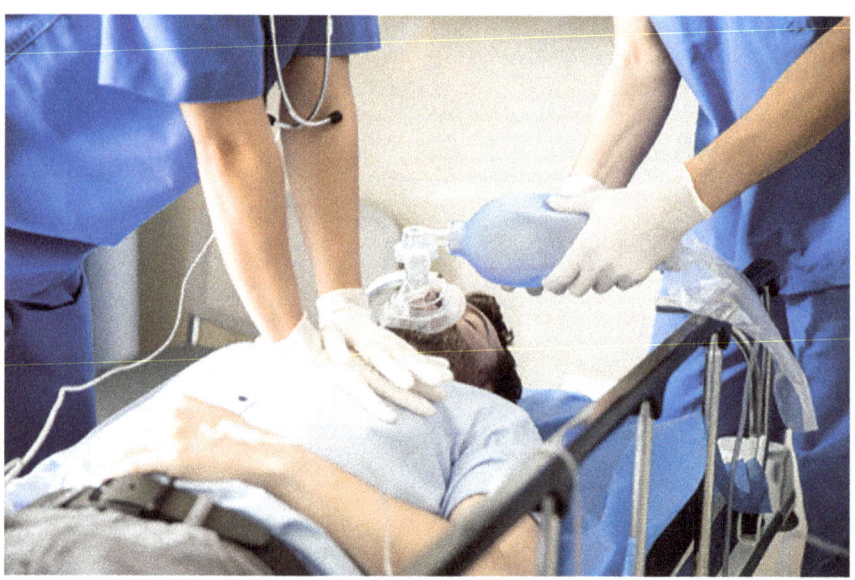

Questions to Ask

1	Who found the patient?
2	What did that person witness?
3	How long has the patient been down, or when was the patient last seen or heard from?
4	Was the patient complaining of anything earlier?
5	Any recent illnesses or recent trauma?
6	What kind of medical history does the patient have?
7	What kind of medicine is the patient taking? Are they compliant?
8	Any allergies?

Roles in a Cardiac Arrest

Compressor	Individual or individuals that are being switched out for chest compressions. Keep an eye on compressor's fatigue. Make sure to switch out often.
AED/monitor/defibrillator	Individual who brings in and operates the monitor. Make sure it's placed in a position where the team leader can see the monitor.
Airway	Individual who opens the airway and provides ventilation and utilizes both BLS and ALS airways if within scope of practice.

Team leader	Every resuscitation must have a team leader. This individual assigns roles to team members and orchestrates the code from start to finish. The team leader also makes the treatment decisions. The team leader also assumes responsibilities for roles that are not assigned.
IV/IO/ medication	An ACLS provider role. This individual initiates IV/IO access and administers medications.
Scribe/timer	Typically, the captain scribes. It is important to have a scribe to keep track of times for CPS and all interventions performed.

Reversible Causes

H	Hypovolemia
H	Hypoxia
H	Hydrogen ion (acidosis)
H	Hypo/hyperkalemia
H	Hypothermia
T	Tension pneumothorax
T	Tamponade cardiac
T	Toxins
T	Thrombosis pulmonary
T	Thrombosis coronary

Treatment (Follow Local Protocols or ACLS)

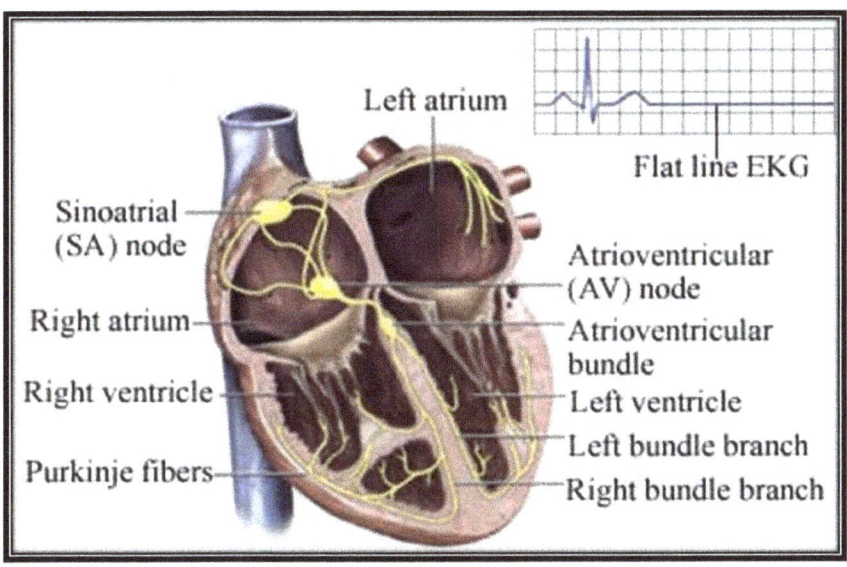

Asystole/PEA (general guide: always use ACLS or follow local protocols)	1. Establish team lead and delegate assignments to team members (see roles in cardiac arrest) and consider delegating someone to gather information. 2. CPR with monitor 3. Airway 4. IV/IO and blood sugar 5. Consider Hs and Ts and treat reversible causes 6. Epinephrine 1:10,000 (1 mg), IV/IO every three minutes
VFIB/VTACH	1. Establish team lead and delegate assignments to team members (see roles in cardiac arrest) and Consider delegating someone to gather information

(general guide: always use ACLS or follow local protocols)	2. CPR with monitor 3. Defibrillate if appropriate 4. airway 5. IV/IO and blood sugar 6. Epinephrine 1:10,000, amiodarone; continue with just epinephrine	
ROSC (general guide: always use ACLS or follow local protocols)	1. Obtain vital signs and treat appropriate rhythm 2. Consider fluid bolus 3. Consider dopamine if fluid bolus is not working 4. Transport code 3 to STEMI/STAR center 5. Consider therapeutic hypothermia if protocol states	

Differential Diagnosis

1	Workable or not workable. (Check death in the field protocol for declaring death in the field.)
2	Trauma. (Follow protocols for traumatic arrest.)
3	Medical. (Treat appropriately.)
4	Crime scene. (Make sure not to disturb evidence.)

Words of Advice

1	As an intern, it can be nerve-racking to run your first couple cardiac arrests. Remember, you are in charge of these calls. When you first show up, introduce yourself as an intern as say you would like to run this code. I recommend working your first cardiac arrest as a team lead to demonstrate that you know how to run a code. This is obviously up to the discretion of your preceptor.
2	Try your best to stay as organized as possible. Make sure you have everyone in an appropriate spot and make sure you have a scribe set up.
3	Remember not to disturb anything after the code is finished.
4	Remember to be sympathetic and understand that people will be upset.
5	Know your local protocols and ACLS.
6	Know what kind of monitor you are using (biphasic or monophasic) and the joules that you will be using.

Chapter 12

TRAUMA

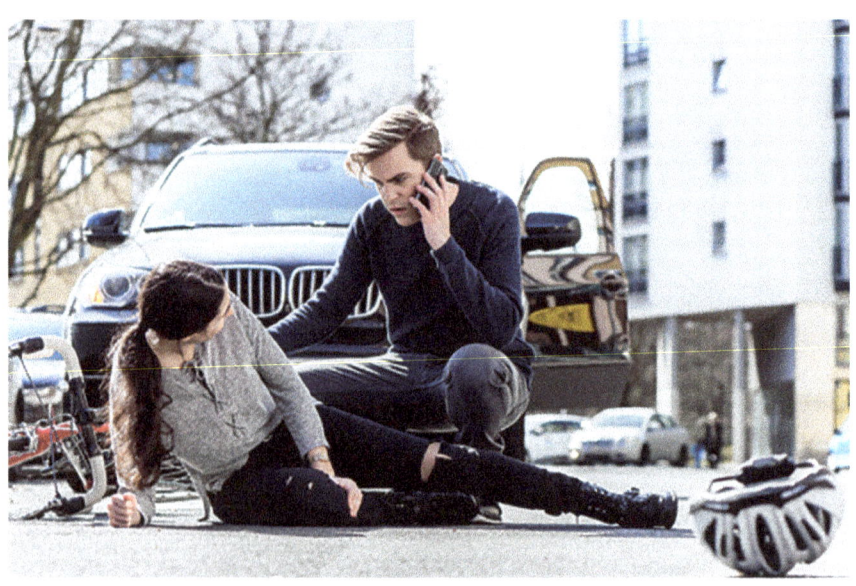

What to Look For

1	Obvious signs of bleeding
2	Entrance and exit wounds
3	DCAPBTLS
4	Things that could have caused any injuries to see how bad the mechanism is
5	Extrication needs
6	Signs of shock pale, cool and diaphoretic
7	Mechanism
8	Environmental dangers

Compensating shock	1. Clammy (pale, cool, and diaphoretic skin) 2. Nausea/vomiting 3. weak, rapid, thready, or absent distal pulses 4. shortness of breath 5. Agitation, anxiety, restlessness, feeling of impending doom 6. Altered mental status 7. Delayed capillary refill
Decompensating shock	1. Hypotension 2. Thready or absent pulses 3. Labored or irregular breathing 4. Ashen, mottled, or cyanotic skin 5. Dilated pupils

Differential Diagnosis

Cardiac tamponade	Muffled heart tones, narrowed pulse pressure
Flail chest	Three or more cracked or broken ribs in two or more places
Tension pneumothorax	JVD, tracheal deviation, weak or absent pulse on one side, hypotension, SOB, diminished or absent lung sounds.
Internal bleeding	Firm, rigid abdomen, bruising to the belly button or flanks
ICP	High blood pressure, bradycardia, irregular respirations, headache, vomiting without nausea, ALOC
Concussion	Headache, ALOC, loss of consciousness, memory loss, vomiting, weakness, agitation
Sucking chest wound	Frothy blood coming from chest wound

Questions to Ask

1	Can the patient tell you what happened? What is their A&O status and GCS score?
2	Is anything hurting the patient? If so, what is hurting? Any distracting injuries?
3	Did the patient lose consciousness? Do they have full recall of the event?

4	Any medical history, medications, or allergies? Any blood thinners?
5	Any chest pain, shortness of breath, nausea, vomiting, diarrhea, headache, dizziness, weakness, or any recent drug or alcohol use?

Chapter 13

FALLS

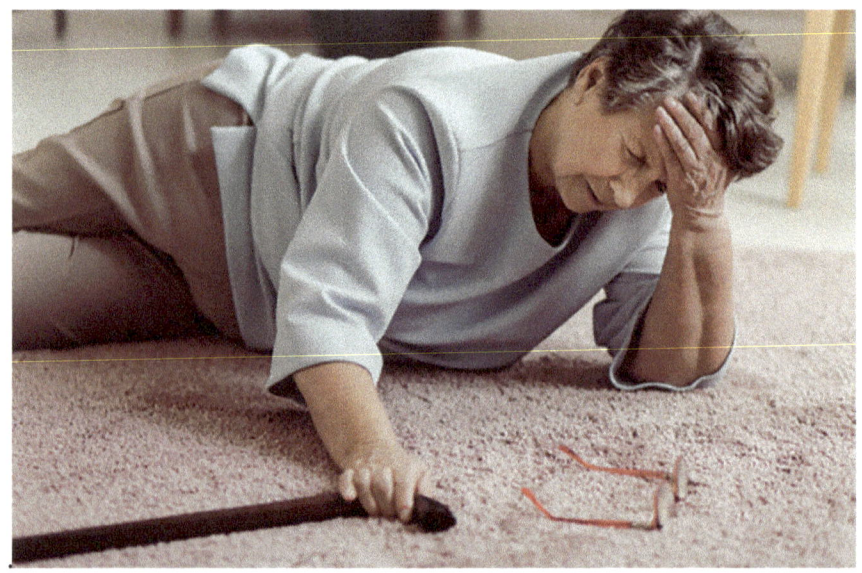

Questions to Ask

1	How did they fall?
2	What position were they in when they fell? Were they standing, sitting, or lying down, riding a bike, skateboarding, etc. when they fell?
3	If the patient was riding a bike, skateboarding, etc., were they wearing a helmet or protection? If so, what kind of damage is on the helmet?
3	What was the height of the fall?
3	What surface did they fall on? Carpet, tile, concrete, or grass?
4	Did the patient hit their head? If so, where?
5	Any loss of consciousness?
6	Any head, neck, or midline back pain? Numbness or tingling to extremities, CSM intact? Assess for C spine.
7	Is the patient taking any blood thinners?
8	What is the patient's mental status? Can they remember what happened before or after the fall?
9	Any dizziness, nausea, vomiting, or blurred vision?
10	Did the patient have any medical complaints before the fall? Remember it could have been due to a seizure, syncope, mechanical fall. Try and determine why the fall happened and make sure to treat any injuries.
12	Are they able to get up? Are they hurting anywhere?
13	How does the patient normally get around? Unassisted, cane, walker, or wheelchair?

14	Has the patient been falling more frequently? Do they have a caretaker? If not, you should recommend the patient to look into a medical alert necklace in case this happens again or possibly recommend a caretaker if they do not already have one if appropriate.
13	Remember your protocols for trauma criteria.

Chapter 14

MOTORIZED VEHICLE ACCIDENT

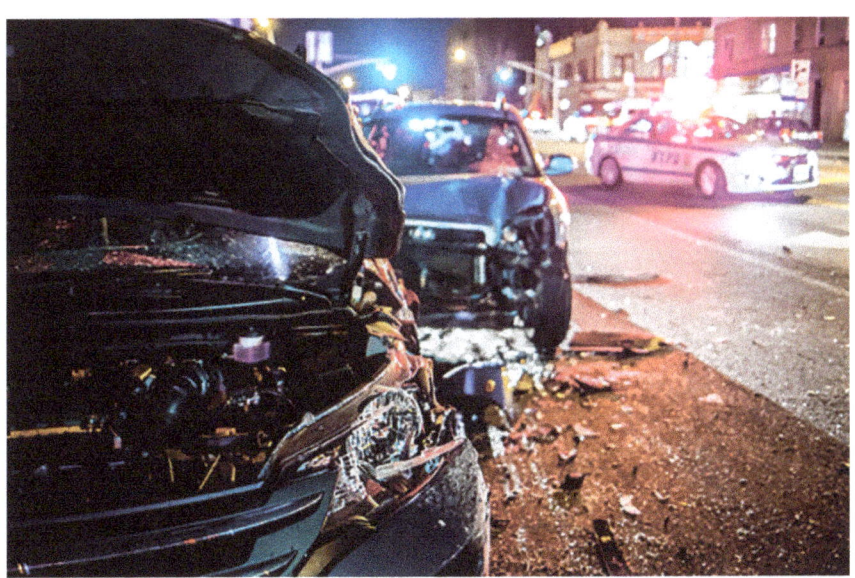

What to Look for and Be Aware Of

1	*Make sure you are aware of your safety on these calls.* Wear something that has high visibility, especially at night. Not all drivers pay attention, and most firstresponders I know have had close calls with being hit by cars. Make sure to always pay attention.
2	As you are approaching the scene, look at how many vehicles are involved. Is this an MCI? Do you need more resources? Traffic control? Additional engines or trucks? A supervisor?
3	What kind of damage do you see on the vehicles? Look for intrusion to the vehicle, airbag deployment, and damage to the windows. Look for starring on the windshield or a bent steering wheel column.
4	What kind of accident was it? T-bone, head-on, rear-ended. Did the car roll over?
5	Do you have any patients that need to be extricated, or have they all been self-extricated?
6	How fast were the vehicles going before the impact? Are there skid marks indicating they attempted to slow down prior to the collision?
7	Were the drivers restrained?
8	Make sure to check C spine early.
9	Are police officers on scene? If people are getting transported, find out if the police officers need any information. If the patient is critical, ask if the police can meet at the hospital?
10	Why did the accident occur? Was the driver intoxicated? If so, find out if they are going to be in custody. Were they distracted?

11	Notice any car seats in the back of any vehicles? Make sure to check for possible ejections from people with no proper seat belts. Make sure all patients are accounted for.
12	Any auto vs. pedestrians?
13	Know your trauma criteria regarding auto accidents.
14	Make sure to delegate on scene. Let other responders know what you needhelp with, whether it is finding out additional information or assessing other patients.
15	If it is a motorcycle accident, was the patient wearing any protection? Helmet, leathers, boots? If so, what is the damage to those?
16	Was the rider separated from the bike?
17	How fast was the rider going?
18	Make sure to do your head-to-toe assessment and assess lung sounds for possibility of a pneumothorax.

Chapter 15

OVERDOSE

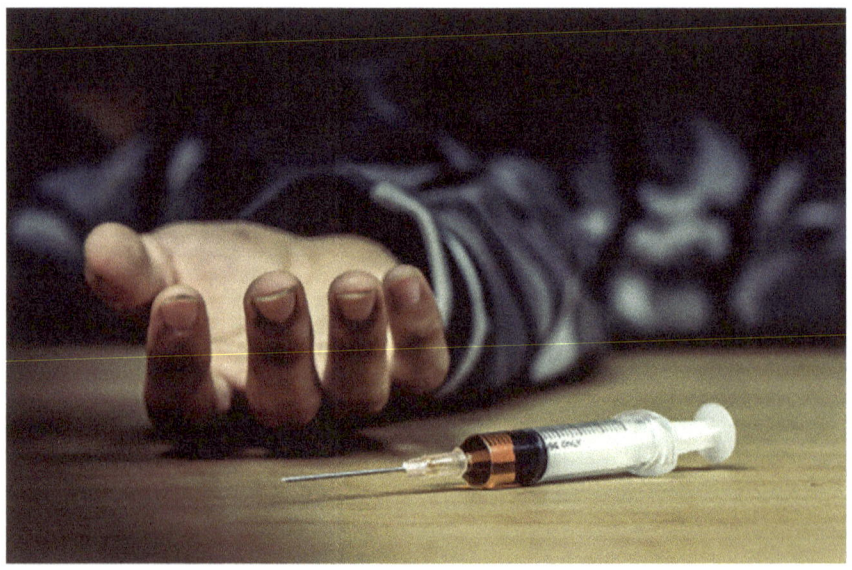

Questions to Ask or Things to Look For

1	Make sure to assess ABCs and treat appropriately.
2	What kind of symptoms is the patient having?
3	What did the patient overdose on? If the patient is altered, check your surroundings. Is there anything the patient could have overdosed on?
4	How much could they have taken? Any empty or full pill bottles?
5	Does the patient have a history of depression or is suicidal?
6	Does the patient want to hurt themselves, hurt others, or is gravely disabled? Are there police officers on scene? Is a 5150 going to be written up?
7	Have they ever overdosed before? Why did they overdose? When did they overdose?
8	Did anything specific happen recently that made them want to overdose?

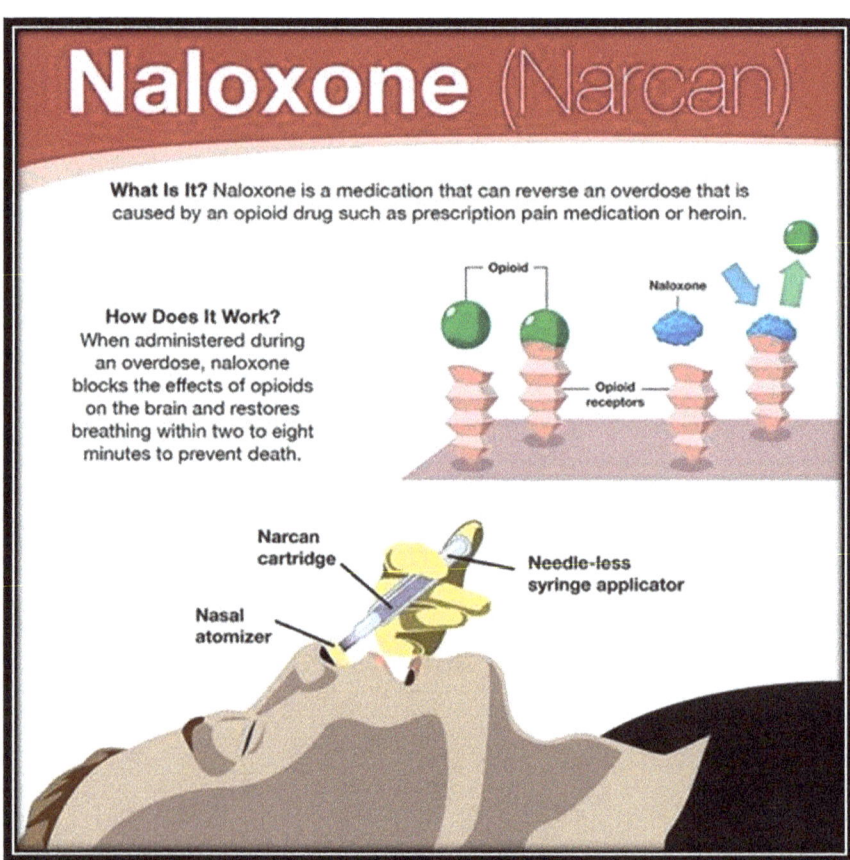

Chapter 16

BEHAVIORAL

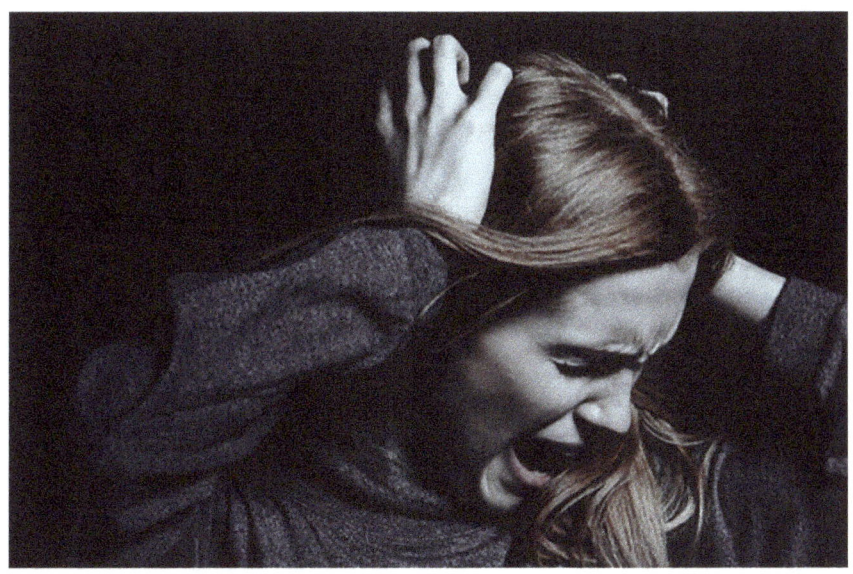

Things to Look for and Ask

1	First of all, make sure you and your partner are safe.
2	What's going on today?
3	What actions or behaviors they are exhibiting?
4	What is their level of consciousness and mental status?
5	Any drug or alcohol use today?
6	What is their medical history? Any psych history, bipolar disorder, schizophrenia?
7	Are they supposed to be taking any medication?
8	Are they compliant with their medication? If not, then why? (A lot of our homeless population gets their drugs stolen on the street.)
9	Any hallucinations or visual disturbances? Are they hearing any voices? What are they seeing? What are those voices telling them?
10	Do they want to hurt themselves or anyone else? Is the patient gravely disabled (5150)?

Words of Wisdom

1	*Safety on these calls is incredibly important.* When people are under the influence of drugs and are have mental illnesses, things can change really quickly. Make sure you and your partner are aware of your patient's body positioning and behavior.
2	If there are any worries about a patient potentially becoming violent, restrain them. Call for assistance if you need to.

3	When administering a sedative such as Midazolam IM, make sure the patient is not moving around. Use multiple people to hold the person down to administer the medication and do so quickly and safely without hesitation. It can be very easy to get a needle stick when a patient is trying to resist your medical care. Be safe.
4	Spit can still go through spit masks. Always wear your eye protection.
5	If your patient starts spitting, and you plan on using spit mask, be careful when you apply it. Patients can bite you.
6	Use gravity to your advantage. It is harder for a patient to get up and try to fight you if they are lying down flat on your gurney and have all the seat belts on.

Differential Diagnosis

Hypoxia	SPO2 < 92
Drugs	Dilated or pinpoint pupils, HX of drug use, track marks, erratic behavior
Hypoglycemia	Blood sugar below sixty
CVA	Chief complaint of a headache prior to your arrival
ETOH	Empty bottles lying around, smells of ETOH, alcohol withdrawal
Head injury	Recent falls, recent trauma to the head, patient may appear combative

Chapter 17

ETOH

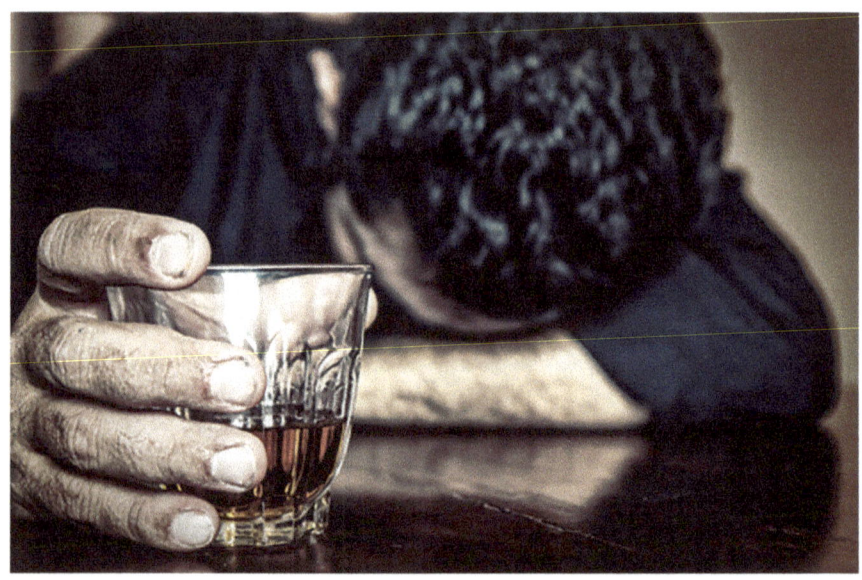

Things to Look For

1	Scene safety
2	Bottles lying around on scene. Look to see if they are empty.
3	Smell of ETOH
4	Incontinence
5	Slurred speech (perform stroke assessment)
6	Signs of any trauma
7	Distended abdomen
8	Engorged liver
9	Wernicke's syndrome (type of brain disorder caused by lack of B-1 vitamin or thiamine. Symptoms may include confusion and changes to the eyes and vision such as a drooping upper eyelid and up-and-down or side-to-side eye movement or double vision and ataxia or loss of muscle coordination (the patient may also hallucinate).

Questions to Ask

1	What have you been drinking today, and how much have you had to drink today?
2	Are you drinking more than usual today?
3	Do you have withdrawals from alcohol?
4	How long does it take without a drink for you to experience your withdrawal symptoms?
5	What happens during your withdrawals?

6	When was your last drink?
7	Are you experiencing withdrawals now?
8	Do you have seizures or any other medical history?

Signs and Symptoms of ETOH

1	Ataxia
2	Incontinence
3	CNS depression
4	Impaired or slurred speech
5	Smells of ETOH
6	Flushed face
7	Red eyes
8	Impaired thinking
9	Memory impairment

Signs and Symptoms of Withdrawal

1	Restlessness, shakiness, sweating, loss of appetite
2	Nausea or vomiting
3	Anxiety or nervousness
4	Tachycardia, tremors, headache, insomnia, disorientation
5	Seizures
6	Agitation or irritability

7	Hypertension
8	Fever

Symptoms and Effects of Alcoholism

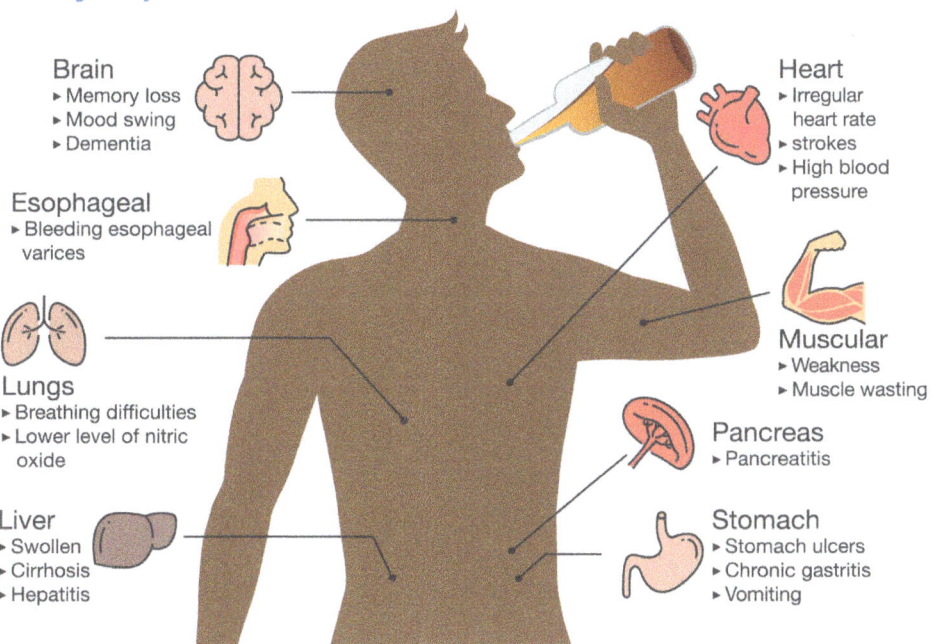

Chapter 18

POISONINGS

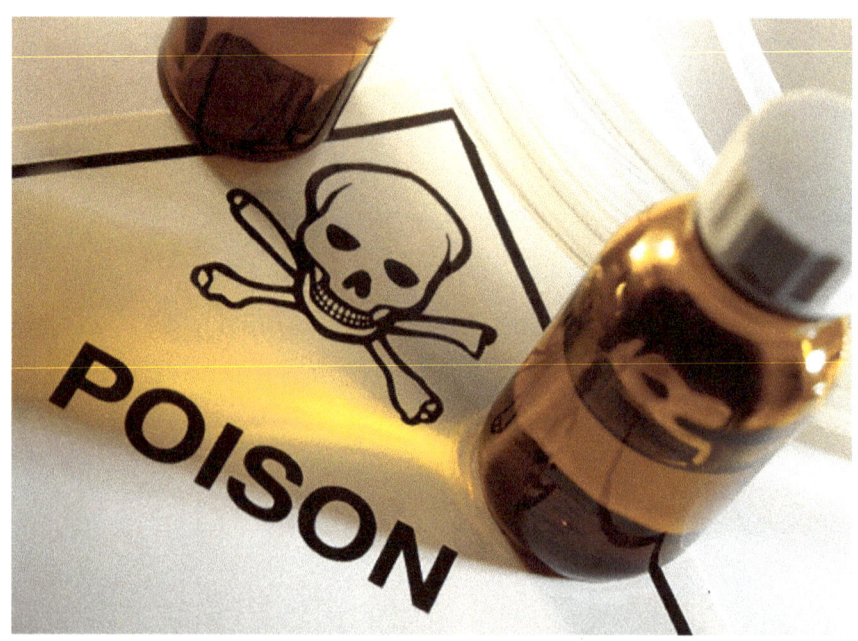

Findings That May Indicate Potential Poisoning

1	Decreased level of consciousness
2	Airway compromise, injuries from chemical burns, edema, mouth full of pills, etc.
3	Abnormal respiratory pattern or potential for atonal respirations
4	Dysrhythmias that affect the heart rate such as tachycardia and bradycardia
5	Combative, intoxication, delirium

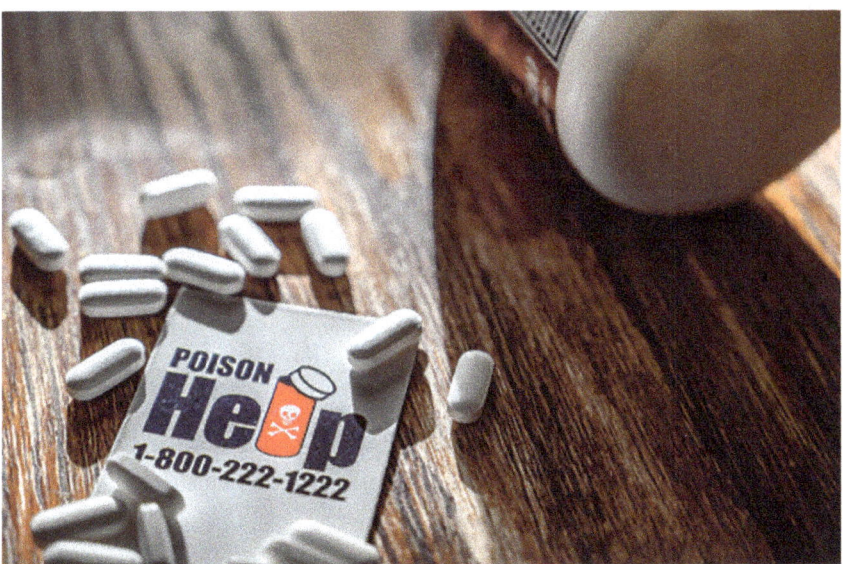

LIST OF ADSORBED TOXINS

Agents WELL Adsorbed by Activated Charcoal

Acetylsalicylic Acid	Chloroquines & Primaquine	Indomethacin & other NSAIDs	Phenylbutazone
Aflatoxin			Phenylpropanolamine
Amphetamines	Cimetidine	Kerosene, Benzene,	Piroxicam
Antidepressants	Dapsone	Dichloroethane	Phenol Syrup of
Antiepileptics	DDT	Malathion & other Pesticides	IPECAC constituents
Antihistamines	Dextropropoxyphene & other opioids	Meprobamate	Quinidine & Quinine
Aspirin/ Other Salicylates	Digitalis	Nefopam	Strychnine
Atropine	DIQUAT & other Herbicides	Methotrexate	Tetracyclines
Barbiturates		Mexiletine	Theophylline
Benzodiazepines	Glycosides Disopyramide	NSAIDS (e.g. Tolfenamin Acid)	Torbutamide, Chlorpropamide
Beta-blockers	Ergot Alkaloids	*Paracetamol	Carbutamide,
Biphenyls	Furosemide	PARAQUAT	Tolazamide
Carbamazepine	Glibenclamide & Glipizide Glutethimide	Polychlorinated Phenothiazines	

Agents POORLY Adsorbed by Activated Charcoal

Cyanide
Ethanol
Ethylene Glycol
Iron
Isopropanol
Lithium
Methanol
Strong Mineral Acids & Alkali

* In cases of severe paracetamol poisoning, concurrent intravenous antidote (N-acetylcysteine) administration and oral Norit Carbomix is recommended.

Try and Determine the Following

Note: activated charcoal should be withheld when the toxic ingestion occurred longer than an hour before EMS arrival.

1	What was the substance that was ingested?
2	When was the substance ingested?
3	How much of the substance was ingested?
4	Was there an attempt to vomit, or did the patient vomit prior to EMS arrival?
5	Has an antidote or activated charcoal or ipecac been administered prior to EMS arrival? (*Remember that a contraindication to activated charcoal is active vomiting.*)
6	Does the patient have any psychiatric history or history of suicide attempts? Any recent depression?

Chapter 19

PAIN MANAGEMENT

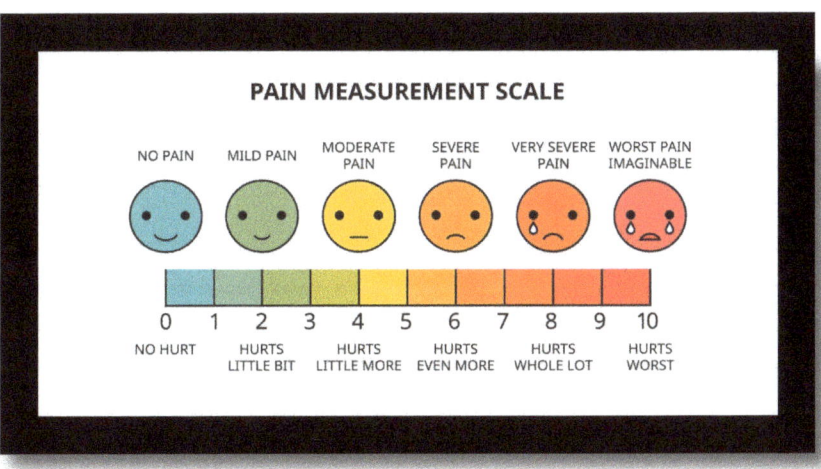

Questions to Ask

1	What happened?
2	When did the pain start? Is it new or chronic?
3	Does anything make the pain better or worse?
4	Can you describe the pain?
5	Does the pain radiate or go anywhere else?
6	How would you rate your pain on a scale from 1–10?
7	Have you prescribed any medication for your pain? Have you taken that medication?
8	Any drug allergies?
9	If it is an extremity injury, are they comfortable in the position they are currently in? Is their injury self-splinted right now? Is it better to let them self-splint or to splint it up yourself?
10	Does that extremity have a pulse? If so, mark the pulse with a pen or marker so it's easy to locate.

Pain Medication from Strongest to Weakest

Fentanyl	Fentanyl is a synthetic opioid that is thirty to fifty times more potent than heroin. Fentanyl is a prescription drug generally prescribed for patients to manage severe pain after surgery. Common brand names for fentanyl include Actiq, Duragesic, and Sublimaze. It may also be prescribed for patients with chronic pain who have built a physical tolerance to other opioids.

	Due to its potency and addictive qualities, fentanyl is a schedule II drug and is considered dangerous. Just a tiny dose of fentanyl can kill a person, about .25 of a milligram.
Heroin	Heroin is the second strongest opioid, a semisynthetic opioid derived from morphine, and a natural substance that comes from the poppy plant. Heroin is the only illegal drug included in this list as most opioids serve a medicinal purpose, whereas heroin does not. Heroin is also the only schedule I drug on the list and has a very strong potential for abuse. It is used by injecting, snorting, or smoking and is often found as a white or black powder or a black sticky substance. When injected, heroin enters the bloodstream and then the brain more rapidly than other opioids, creating immediate feelings of euphoria.
Hydromorphone	Hydromorphone is another strong opioid that is two to eight times more potent than morphine. Prescribed as a severe pain reliever in the brand name Dilaudid, hydromorphone produces feelings of sedation and relaxation. Hydromorphone is a schedule II drug with high potential for abuse, likely leading to physical and psychological dependence. It is commonly abused as a substitute for heroin because it can be dissolved in liquid and injected into the bloodstream to experience the effects faster.

Oxymorphone	Although fourth on the list, oxymorphone is a very strong opioid. Found in the brand name Opana, oxymorphone is prescribed to treat moderate to severe pain. It generally comes in tablet form but is sometimes prescribed as an injectable solution. Oxymorphone is a schedule II opioid with potential for both abuse and dependence. It is abused by oral ingestion, snorting, and injection and can be illegally bought off the street, acquired through forged prescriptions, or stolen during pharmaceutical robberies.
Methadone	While methadone is used under strict medical supervision to treat addiction or painful symptoms of withdrawal, nonmedical use is illegal. Methadone is chemically dissimilar to heroin and morphine but still produces similar effects of euphoria and sedation. Methadone is a schedule II drug and, when abused, can lead to physical and psychological dependence. Swallowed as a tablet or injected as a liquid, methadone abuse can produce adverse health effects if not administered under careful medical supervision.
Oxycodone	While oxycodone is not as strong as the above opioids, it is still considered a schedule II drug with high potential for abuse and dependence. Found in brand names Oxycontin, Roxicodone, and Percocet, oxycodone is generally prescribed to relieve moderate to moderately severe pain. Oxycodone is routinely prescribed in the US and has been abused since the 1960s for its sedating and calming effects.

Morphine	Morphine is the only natural opiate (non-synthetic opioid) on the list but is included because the potency of opioids is often compared to morphine. Often prescribed to treat pain when other opioids are ineffective, morphine is similar in potency to oxycodone. Morphine is a schedule-II-controlled substance and was traditionally misused as an injectable liquid but can now be administered as oral solutions and ingestible tablets. Injecting morphine is usually preferred as it enters the bloodstream and reaches the brain more quickly.
Hydrocodone	Hydrocodone is near equipotent to morphine and is generally prescribed to treat moderate pain. Some brand names for hydrocodone include Vicodin, Lortab, and Hycodan. More potent than codeine, hydrocodone is the most frequently prescribed opioid in the US with a staggering 136 million prescriptions filled in the first several months of 2014. Hydrocodone is a schedule II drug commonly abused with alcohol. A 2013 survey found that over twenty-four million people over the age of 12 had taken hydrocodone for no medical reason. Hydrocodone is a good example of how a weaker opioid can be abused and pose serious health risks; in 2011, over 82,000 emergency room visits were attributed to hydrocodone.
Codeine	Codeine is weaker in potency and is generally prescribed to treat mild to moderate pain and may be used with other medications to reduce coughing.

	Depending on which drug it is combined with, codeine is either a schedule II, III, or V drug. Schedule II codeine is found in some forms of morphine. Other prescriptions, like Tylenol with codeine, are schedule III and are stronger than cough medicines that contain less than 200 mg of codeine (schedule V).
Meperidine	Meperidine, brand name Demerol, was the first synthetic opioid ever created. Meperidine is weaker than most other opioids but is still considered a schedule II drug because of the potential for abuse. Physical dependence and tolerance are likely to develop quicker than most opioids, making abuse of this drug as dangerous as any opioid. Although, meperidine is considered medically ineffective compared to other opioids.
Tramadol	Tramadol has similar potency to meperidine but, as a schedule IV drug, has less potential for physical dependence, tolerance, and abuse. However, tramadol, or brand name Ultram, can still be abused by those suffering from addiction or chronic pain. In 2012, 3.2 million people reported having used tramadol for nonmedical purposes. Although tramadol is the weakest opioid on the list, it is still commonly abused and can lead to addiction.

Medications with Few Side Effects *(for Mild to Moderate Pain)*			
Name	**Active Ingredient**	**Side Effects**	**Administration**
Tylenol	Acetaminophen	None	Pills, liquid or IV
Motrin	Ibuprofen	Some stomach discomfort	Pills, liquid or IV
Aleve	Naproxen	Some stomach discomfort	Pills
Medications with Some Side Effects *(for Mild, Moderate or Sevre Pain)*			
Toradol	Ketorolac	Mild bleeding risk	Pills or IV
Neurontin	Gabapentin	Sedation	Pills
Lyrica	Pregabalin	Sedation	Pills
Local Anesthetics	Lidocaine, bupivacaine, ropivacaine	Numbness	Injection or patch
Steroids	Dexamethasone, hydrocortisone	Can increase glucose levels in diabetics	Pills or IV
Aspirin	Acetylsalicylic acid	Some stomach discomfort, easy bruising or bleeding	Pills
Medications with More Side Effects *(for Severe Pain)*			
Morphine	Morphine	Constipation, dizziness, sleepiness, nervousness, nauseous	Pills, liquid, IV or IV patient-controlled

Dilaudid	Hydromorphone	Constipation, dizziness, sleepiness, nervousness, nauseous	Pills, liquid, IV or IV patient-controlled
Fentanyl	Fentanyl	Constipation, dizziness, sleepiness, nervousness, nauseous, problems breathing	IV or patch
Vicodin/ Lortab/ Norco	Hydrocodone/ acetaminophen	Constipation, dizziness, sleepiness, nervousness, nauseous	Pills
Percocet	Oxycodone/ acetaminophen	Constipation, dizziness, sleepiness, nervousness, nauseous	Pills

Chapter 20

PREGNANCY

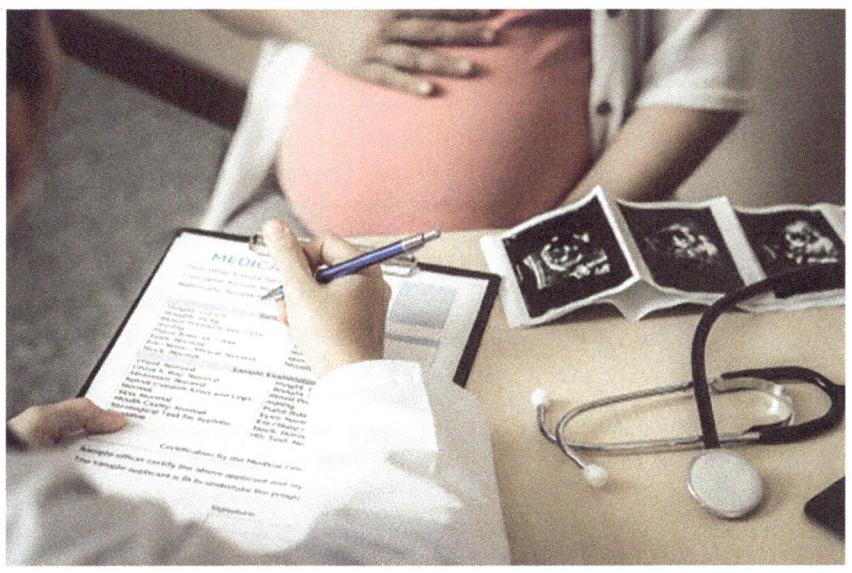

Pregnancy Trimesters

Questions to Ask

1	How far along is their pregnancy? When is their due date?
2	How many times have they been pregnant?
3	How many times have they given birth? Any complications during those births?
4	Has the patient's water broken or any bleeding or unusual vaginal discharge?
5	Have they seen a doctor? Are there any expected complications?
6	Is the patient experiencing any contractions? If so, how far apart are they?
7	Do they feel the urge to push or bear down? If so, check for crowning.
8	What hospital are they supposed to deliver at?
9	Any recent trauma or illnesses?
10	Any medical history, allergies, or medications?

Key Terms

Ectopic pregnancy	This occurs when a fertilized ovum is implanted outside of the endometrial lining of the uterine wall.
Gravida	The number of times a patient has been pregnant.
Parity	The number of live births.
Placenta previa	A condition that occurs when the placenta partially or totally obstructs the cervix.
Placenta abruption	Occurs when the placenta or a portion of it tears away from the inner lining of the uterus.
Spontaneous abortion (miscarriage)	Death of the fetus prior to twenty weeks gestation absent outside intervention.

Key Anatomy

Amniotic sac	The membranous sac filled with amniotic fluid that surrounds the fetus during development.
Cervix	The lower, narrow portion of the uterus.
Placenta	The organ that provides oxygen and nourishment to the fetus during fetal development.
Uterus	The pouch-like structure where the fertilized ovum is implanted and the fetus develops.

Pregnancy Complications

Ectopic pregnancy	An ectopic pregnancy occurs when a fertilized ovum is implanted outside of the endometrial lining of the uterine wall. While the site of improper implantation can vary, it most often occurs within the fallopian tubes. As the ovum begins to develop into an embryo and eventually into a fetus, it will stretch the fallopian tube, which can result in rupture and massive hemorrhage. Any woman of childbearing years who presents with abdominal pain is considered to have an ectopic pregnancy until proven otherwise by hospital staff. Typically occurs at the seven- to eight-week mark in the pregnancy.
Placenta previa	A medical condition that occurs when the entire placenta or a portion of it covers the opening to the cervix. This condition is important for EMS professionals to recognize because it may prevent the ability for the baby tobe delivered vaginally, which increases the urgency to rapidly recognize the condition and quickly transport the patient. If the patient has been going to her doctor's appointments, the patient should already know that they have the placenta covering the opening of the cervix.

Placenta abruption	Occurs when a portion or the entire placenta detaches from the uterine wall prior to birth. This condition complicates approximately 1 percent of all pregnancies. The detachment can cause significant bleeding that can be concealed such as when the bleeding accumulates behind the placenta. It's also possible for the patient to experience vaginal bleeding. Because the detachment is not due to the natural process of birth, abdominal pain is a common presenting symptom.
Spontaneous abortion	Commonly called a miscarriage, it is defined as fetal death prior to twenty weeks gestation that is not due to medical intervention. EMS providers can expect to be called to this type of pregnancy complication because it is present in up to 20 percent of recognized pregnancies. In most cases, the primary focus for EMS providers is toprovide psychological support to the female patient and family. The patient does not often present with an acute condition. If the patient has passed fetal tissue, collect all parts for examination by a physician. Transport to the hospital is necessary because the patient will require follow-up care to ensure that no fetal parts remain.

Gestational diabetes	A female who was not diabetic before pregnancy can develop what is known as gestational diabetes. This condition affects approximately 18 percent of all pregnancies. A screening test, known as a glucose screening test or glucose tolerance test, is administered to the expectant mother when she seeks prenatal care. If the test is positive, the more definitive "glucose tolerance test" is used to make the diagnosis. Since insulin does not cross the placenta, but glucose does, the excess glucose levels in the mother's bloodstream result in an increase in calories for the fetus. A mother seeking prenatal care will be coached on how to check and control her blood sugar level. *Patients whose mothers have gestational diabetes tend to be larger, which can lead to delivery complications.* *Make sure to check your blood sugar.*
Preeclampsia and eclampsia	Hypertension in pregnancy can be a serious concern, and a recent study found that the number of delivery hospitalizations in the US with hypertensive disorders in pregnancy is increasing. A blood pressure greater than 140/90 mmHg is considered abnormal for the pregnant patient. If the patient is found to have elevated blood pressure, protein in the urine, edema, and is beyond twenty weeks of gestation, she is diagnosed with preeclampsia. This condition typically takes place during the first pregnancy and occurs more frequently and severely in women who are pregnant with more than one fetus, have chronic hypertension, previously had preeclampsia, were diabetic

before the pregnancy, or had thrombophilia (increased tendency to form clots).

Eclampsia is defined as a seizure occurring during pregnancy when there is no other known cause (i.e., it is not epilepsy or other identifiable cause). Twenty-five percent of the seizures occur before labor, 50 percent during labor, and 25 percent after delivery, which can occur as much as ten days after delivery.

Typically treated in the field with magnesium sulfate.

Chapter 21

CHILDBIRTH

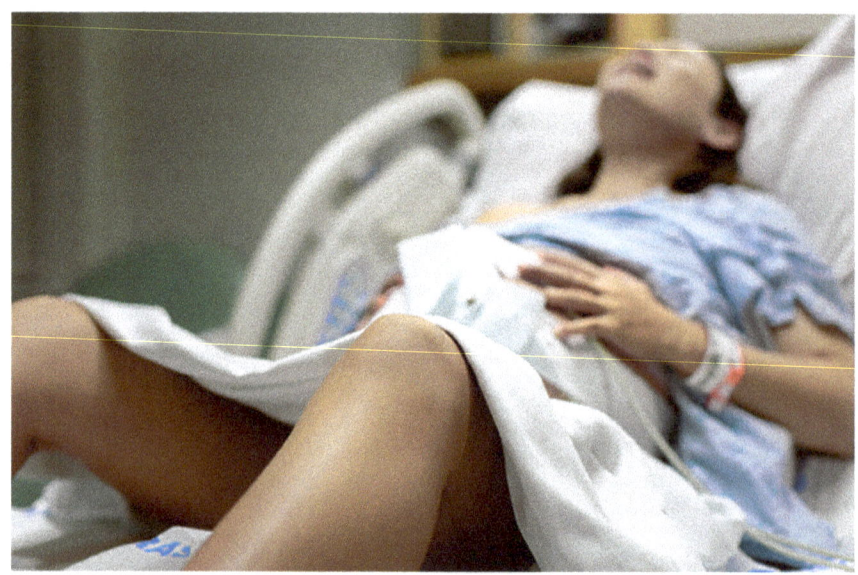

Questions to Ask

1	How far along is their pregnancy? When is their due date?
2	How many times have they been pregnant?
3	How many times have they given birth? Any complications during those births?
4	Has the patient's water broken or any bleeding or unusual vaginal discharge?
5	Have you seen a doctor? Are there any expected complications?
6	Is the patient experiencing any contractions? If so, how far apart are they?
7	Do they feel the urge to push or bear down? If so, check for crowning.
8	What hospital are they supposed to deliver at?
9	Any recent trauma or illnesses?
10	Any medical history, allergies, or medications?

STAGES OF BIRTH IN VAGINAL DELIVERY

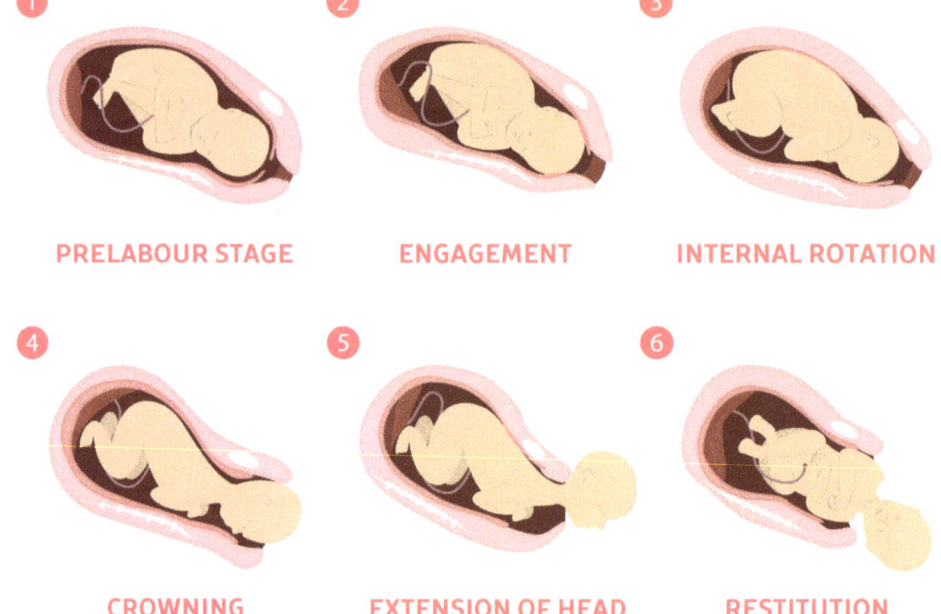

The Stages of Labor/Delivery

Labor Stages

Stage 1	*Dilation*—regular contractions, thinning, and gradual dilation of cervix; ends with fully dilated cervix (10 cm). Lasts twelve to sixteen hours, primipara; five to seven hours, multipara.
Stage 2	*Expulsion*—fully dilated; the time from when the baby enters the birth canal until he is born. Stage lasts eighty minutes for primipara and thirty minutes for multipara

| Stage 3 | *Placenta delivery*—the time between birth and afterbirth; average time of five to thirty minutes.
"Bloody show" begins with the loss of the mucus plug and continues throughout the delivery. |

Contractions occurring within two minutes of each other should alert you that delivery is imminent.

Consider transporting the mother if delivery does not occur within twenty minutes of experiencing contractions that are two to three minutes apart.

Presentations That Can and Cannot Be Delivered in the Field

Can be delivered	Can't be delivered
- Normal cephalic delivery (headfirst) - Umbilical cord around the neck shoulder - Dystocia - Butt first - Double footling	- Single limb presentation - Prolapsed umbilical cord

Childbirth Delivery Instructions

The Stages of Labor & Birth in a Vaginal Delivery

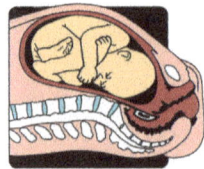

Head Floating Before Engagement
❶

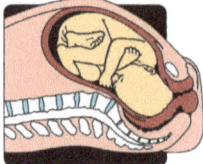

Engagement, Flexion, Descent
❷

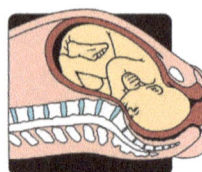

Further Descent, Internal Rotation
❸

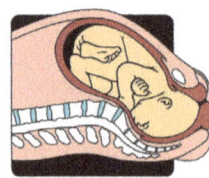

Complete Rotation, Beginning Extension
❹

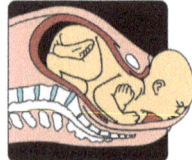

Complete Extension
❺

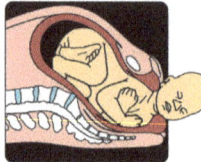

Restitution (External Rotation)
❻

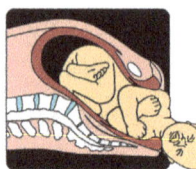

Delivery of Anterior Shoulder
❼

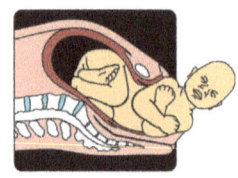

Delivery of Posterior Shoulder
❽

1	*Encourage the mother to breathe deeply between contractions and to push with contractions.*
2	As the baby's head crowns, support it with gentle pressure over the perineum and gently support their head as the head delivers to avoid an explosive birth and prevent injury.
3	If the amniotic sac is still intact, rupture it with a finger to allow amniotic fluid to leak out. Note the color and character of the amniotic fluid: normal fluid is clear or straw-colored; meconium in the fluid produces a tainted, discolored, thick, pea-soup-like color and should be recorded and kept.

4	As soon as the baby's head appears, suction the mouth and nostrils with a bulb syringe. Squeeze air from the syringe before inserting and insert the syringe no more than one inch into the mouth and no more than half an inch into each nostril. *Note: If you see signs of meconium staining, do not stimulate the infant before suctioning the mouth and nose. This is to avoid aspiration of fecal material that can cause pneumonia.*
5	If the umbilical cord is wrapped around the baby's neck, gently slip it over the head. *Do not force it!* If the cord is too tight to slip over the head, apply umbilical cord clamps and cut the cord. *Note: clamp and cut the umbilical cord only if the baby's head has emerged and is in a position that lows you to manage the airway.*
6	Encourage the mother to push. Support the baby's head as it delivers. Caution, babies are slippery!
7	Let the baby come at its own rate. The only intervention that you may be required to do is to gently pull the baby's shoulders down (one at a time) so that it can squeeze through the vaginal opening; however, this shouldn't be required during a normal birth. To assist in the delivery of the anterior shoulder, apply gentle downward pressure on the shoulder while continually supporting the newborn's head.
8	As soon as the anterior shoulder has delivered, apply gentle upward pressure to assist in the delivery of the posterior shoulder.
9	Once both shoulders have delivered, be ready for the remainder of the body to deliver quickly. Newborn babies are slippery, so handle carefully.

10	Stimulate the newborn to breathe by tapping the feet, if necessary.
11	Once pulsations have stopped, clamp the cord by placing a clamp approximately eight to ten inches from the baby. Place a second clamp approximately two inches from the first, then cut the cord between the clamps. Do not cut or clamp a cord that is still pulsating. Apply one clamp or tie about ten inches from the baby. This leaves enough cord for paramedics and hospital staff to start IV lines. *Note: do not tie, clamp, or cut an umbilical cord on a baby who is not breathing unless the cord is around the baby's neck.*
12	Suction the baby's mouth and nostrils again if the newborn is not breathing or is having respiratory distress.
13	Dry and wrap the baby in a warm blanket and cover its head. One of the greatest risks to a newborn baby is to become hypothermic and hypoglycemic as it attempts to keep warm.
14	Place the newborn on its side to facilitate drainage of secretions.
15	Perform an APGAR assessment at one minute and five minutes after delivery.

Normal Vital Signs For **Newborns**

Temperature	Able to maintain stable body temperature in normal room environment
Pulse	Normally *120 to 160 beats per minute* in the newborn period
Respiratory rate	Normally *forty to sixty breaths per minute* in the newborn period

Apgar Scoring System

	Indicator	0 Points	1 Point	2 Points
A	Activity (muscle tone)	Absent	Flexed arms and legs	Active
P	Pulse	Absent	Below 100 bpm	Over 100 bpm
G	Grimace (reflex irritability)	Floppy	Minimal response to stimulation	Prompt response to stimulation
A	Appearance (skin color)	Blue; pale	Pink body, Blue extremities	Pink
R	Respiration	Absent	Slow and irregular	Vigorous cry

Care of Newborn After delivery

The baby should start to breathe on their own in a couple of seconds.

If breathing does not start spontaneously, you must stimulate it to begin by rubbing the newborn's back or tapping your fingers on the soles of its feet. If the newborn does not start breathing effectively within ten to fifteen seconds of stimulation, use an infant BVM to deliver *gentle puffs* of air, just enough to cause the chest to rise. If there is no response after thirty seconds of assisted ventilation, and the heart rate is less than sixty beats per minute, begin CPR

Keep the newborn warm by drying it and then wrapping it in warmed blankets. After the umbilical cord is clamped and cut, cover the baby's head to maintain body heat. Repeat suctioning of the nose and mouth, if needed.

Place the wrapped baby on the mother's chest for warmth and encourage the mother to breastfeed during transport. Prepare for the delivery of the placenta about twenty minutes after the newborn is delivered.

It is important to realize that the mother may be the more serious patient following a normal delivery. *Postpartum hemorrhage can kill. Fundal massage over the mother's uterus can help stop postpartum bleeding.*

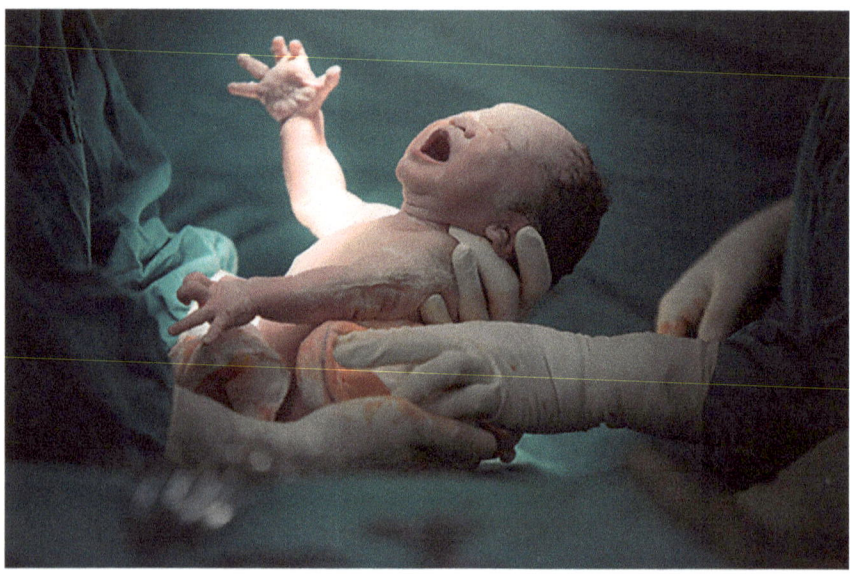

Chapter 22

PEDIATRICS

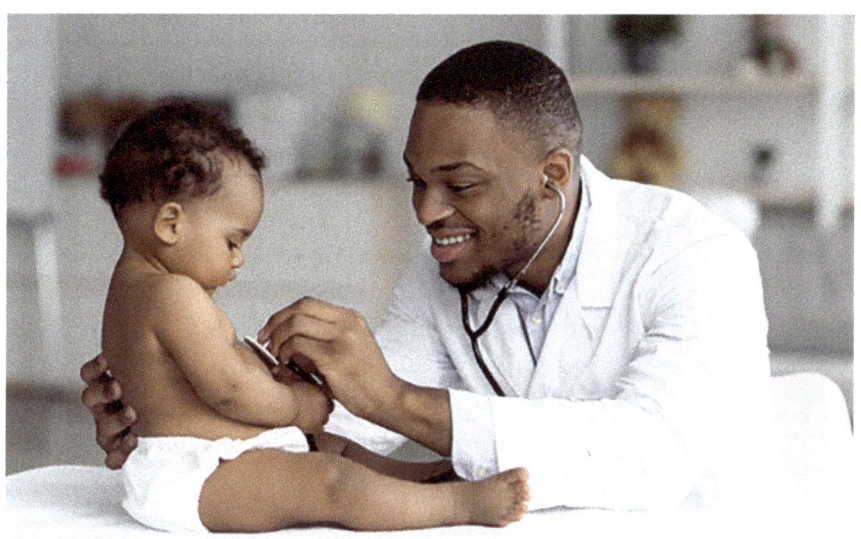

Childhood Development by Age

Infants (zero–one month)	Infants are generally respond to the voice or face of their parents, like to be held by caregivers, and crying can indicate pain, discomfort, or hunger.
Toddlers (one–three years)	Toddlers are curious and, therefore, more apt to have an ingestion emergency or foreign body airway obstruction. Toddlers fear separation from their parents, so giving them a stuffed animal and allowingthem to sit on their parent's lap might help build trust.
Preschoolers (three–five years)	Preschoolers can talk with simple words but often can't understand what's happening and are scared by the sight of blood, so it's important to bandage even the simplest cuts and give constant reassurance.
School-age kids (six–twelve years)	In this age, they can generally answer questions and follow the guidance of EMS providers but have very vivid imaginations, especially about death, and might need constant reminders that they will be okay.
Adolescents (thirteen–eighteen years)	At this age, they can provide accurate information but fear permanent scaring with trauma, and feeling modest is very important to them and can get caught up in the hysteria of a 911 call, so it is important to be well versed in a variety of calming measures.

General Vital Signs and Guidelines

Age	Heart Rate (beats/min)	Blood Pressure (mmHg)	Respiratory Rate (breaths/min)
Premature	110-170	SBP 55-75 DBP 35-45	40-70
0-3 months	110-160	SBP 65-85 DBP 45-55	35-55
3-6 months	110-160	SBP 70-90 DBP 50-65	30-45
6-12 months	90-160	SBP 80-100 DBP 55-65	22-38
1-3 years	80-150	SBP 90-105 DBP 55-70	22-30
3-6 years	70-120	SBP 95-110 DBP 60-75	20-24
6-12 years	60-110	SBP 100-120 DBP 60-75	16-22
> 12 years	60-100	SBP 110-135 DBP 65-85	12-20

Note that all vital signs change with age. I personally keep a pediatric vital sign reference chart in my pocket, which is something you can take a quick glance at. Pediatric calls tend to happen less often. In fact, a recent study showed that more than 54 percent of first responders see zero to one sick child per month.

This means that chances for mistakes are *high*.

Mnemonic for Pediatric Assessment

When you are conducting a primary and secondary assessment in a sick child, the following mnemonic provides a bit more detail than the traditional ABCs, highlights common pediatric-specific considerations, and ensures steps are not missed in the examination:

Airway	Patency, positioning, breath sounds, obstruction
Breathing	Work of breathing, nasal flaring, grunting
Circulation	Heart rate, perfusion, pulses, skin temperature
Disability	Level of consciousness, response to environment
Remove	Remove all clothing and diapers (look for any rashes)

Fahrenheit	Determine body temperatures (hot, normal, cold)
Get	Temperature, pulse, respiratory rate, weight, blood pressure
Head	Head-to-toe exam and history
Inspect	Inspect for evidence of trauma or signs of illness or possible abuse

Remember That Children Compensate Better Than Adults

It is often difficult to predict the severity of illness in a pediatric patient early in an injury or disease process, making it important for EMS providers to understand the compensatory mechanism variations between the adult and child.

There are several distinctions between the adult and pediatric cardiovascular systems. First is that the adult heart increases stroke volume by increasing inotropy (strength of contraction) and chronotropy (rate of contraction) when the stroke volume decreases.

In contrast, the pediatric heart can only increase chronotropy. The pediatric heart has a low compliance as it relates to volume and, therefore, cannot compensate by increasing stroke volume. Consequently, heart rate should be seen as a significant clinical marker when monitoring cardiac output in children. When the pediatric patient becomes bradycardic, it should be assumed that cardiac output has been drastically reduced.

Children rely heavily on the rate of respiration to compensate for respiratory difficulty. Hypoxia is the leading cause of cardiac arrest in pediatric patients.

This is because they are unable to increase the depth of respiration due to the inability of the diaphragm to move farther downward against the compacted abdominal organs.

Conversely, adults can increase the rate and depth of respiration when they experience respiratory difficulty.

Bearing these variations in mind, you should be able to effectively predict when a sick child becomes a critical child.

Pediatric Drug Tricks

These drug tricks were provided by Paramedic Scott Wagness of the SFFD. This not my work.

Adenosine (.033 cc/kg)	To get mg: Take weight and move the decimal over once: 15 kg, 1.5 mg. To get ml: Take the weight in kg and multiply the weight by three then round up to the next highest tenth of an ml. After rounding up, move the decimal over twice: 15kg 15 × 3 = 45, then round up to 50 then move decimal twice .50 = 0.5ml *(Note: for some reason, this doesn't work for 7 kg only. If 7 kg is multiplied by three, then round down to 2 ml.)*
Amiodarone (.1 cc/kg)	To get ml: Move decimal over once: 15 kg = 1.5 ml.
Atropine (.2 cc/kg)	Double the ml and double the mg as epinephrine 1:10,000.

Dextrose 25% D25 (2cc/kg) Dextrose 10% d10w Neonates < 1 month (2 cc/kg) Children > 1 month (5 cc/kg)	To get ml: Double weight 15 kg × 2 = 30 ml D25 To get g: Half weight 15 kg / 2 = 7.5g D25 *Note that this is for D25, not D10!*
Benadryl (.02 cc/kg)	*Mg is same as weight*: 15 kg = 15 mg To get ml: Double weight and move decimal twice. 15 kg × 2 = 30 Move decimal twice: .30 = 0.3 ml.
Epinephrine 1:10,000 (.1cc/kg)	To get ml: Every 10 kg = 1 ml or move decimal over once: 15 kg = 1.5 ml. To get mg: Take ml dose and move decimal over once more 1.5 ml = .15 mg.
Epinephrine 1:1000 (.01cc/kg)	To get ml and mg: Move decimal over twice: 15 kg = .15 mg. 0.15 mg = 0.15 ml

Versed (.02cc/kg)	To get mg: Move decimal once: 15 kg = 1.5 mg. To get ml: Double ml dose and move decimal once more: 1.5 x 2 = 3.0. 0.3 = 0.3 ml
Morphine Greater than six months old (0.1 cc/kg) Less than six months old (.005 cc/kg)	To get mg: Move decimal once 15 kg = 1.5 mg. To get ml: Move decimal once more 1.5 mg = 0.15 ml.
Zofran (every 2 kg = .1cc)	To get mg: Move decimal over once: 15 kg = 1.5 mg. To get ml: Half weight then move decimal once: 15 kg / 2 = 7.5. Move decimal once more = 0.75 ml.

Chapter 23

SEPSIS

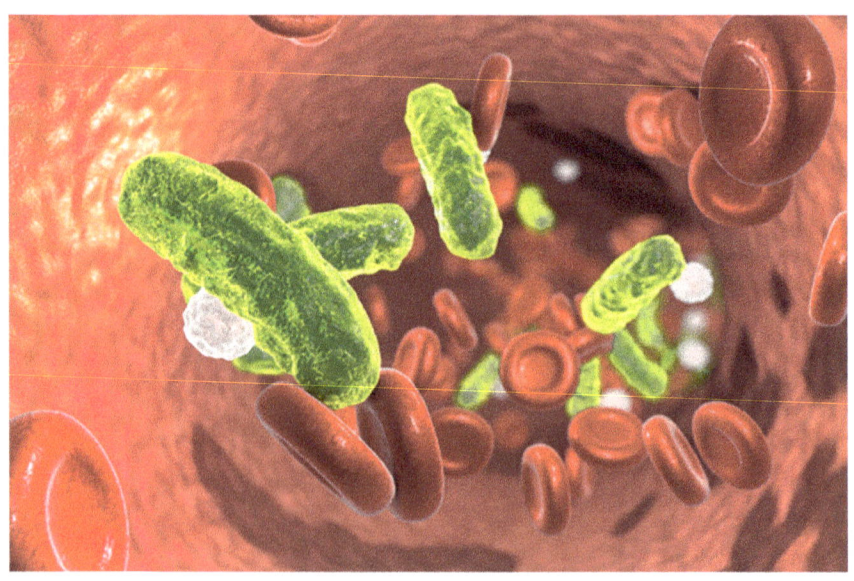

What Is Sepsis?

Sepsis is a potentially life-threatening complication of an infection. Sepsis occurs when chemicals released into the bloodstream to fight the infection trigger inflammatory responses throughout the body. This inflammation can trigger a cascade of changes that can damage multiple organ systems, causing them to fail.

If sepsis progresses to septic shock, blood pressure drops dramatically, which may lead to death.

Anyone can develop sepsis, but it is most common and most dangerous in older adults or those with weakened immune systems. *Early treatment of sepsis, usually with antibiotics and large amounts of intravenous fluids, improves chances for survival.*

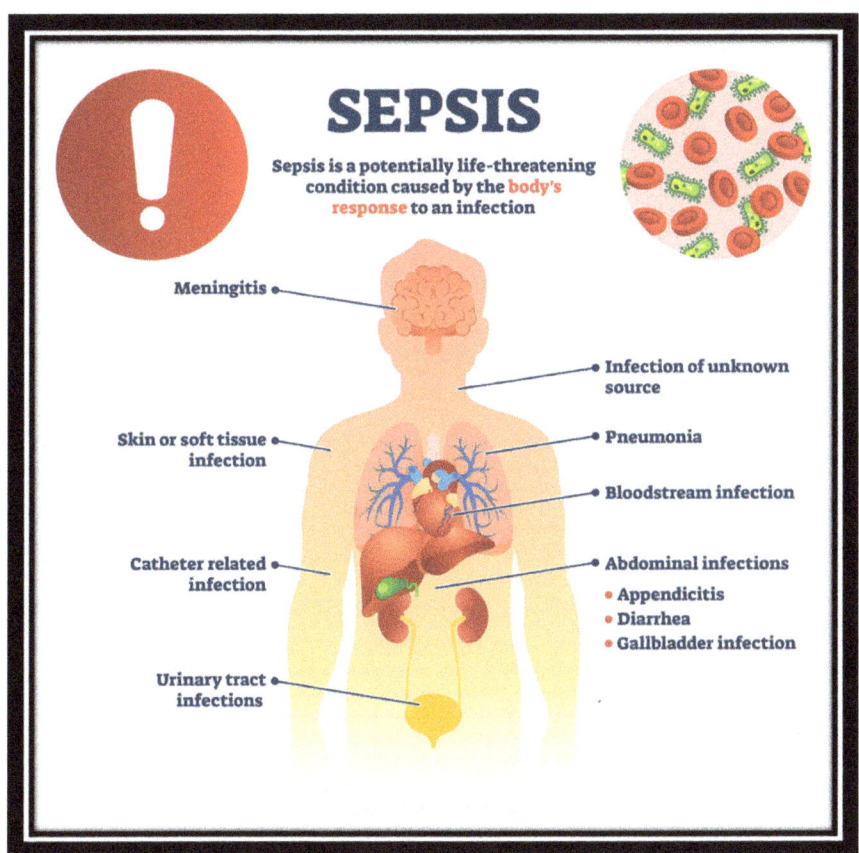

Sepsis Symptoms

Many doctors view sepsis as a three-stage syndrome, starting with sepsis and progressing through severe sepsis to septic shock. The goal is to treat sepsis during its early stage before it becomes more dangerous.

To be diagnosed with sepsis, you must exhibit at least two of these following symptoms plus a confirmed infection:

1	Body temperature above 101 F (38.3 C) or below 96.8 F (36 C)
2	Heart rate higher than ninety beats a minute
3	Respiratory rate higher than twenty breaths a minute

Your diagnosis will be upgraded to severe sepsis if you also exhibit at least one of the following signs and symptoms, which indicate an organ may be failing

Severe Sepsis

1	Significantly decreased urine output
2	Abrupt change in mental status
3	Decrease in platelet count
4	Difficulty breathing
5	Abnormal heart pumping function
6	Abdominal pain

Septic Shock

1	To be diagnosed with septic shock, you must have the signs and symptoms of severe sepsis plus extremely low bloodpressure that does not adequately respondto simple fluid replacement.

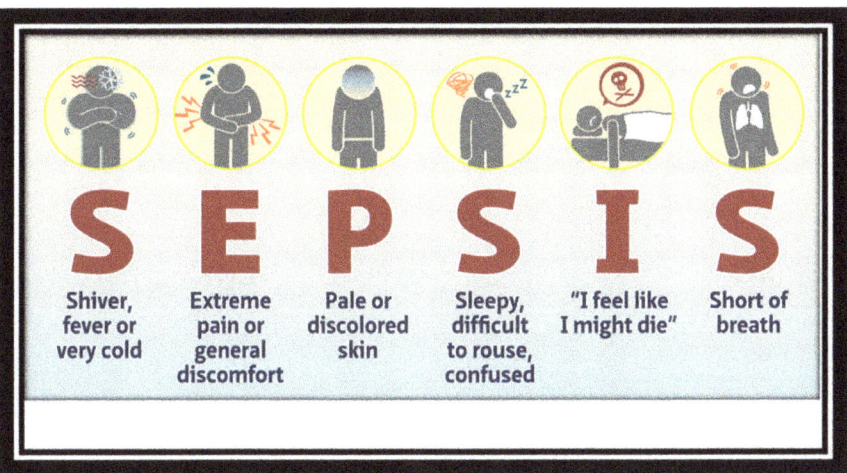

Possible Causes of Sepsis

1	*Remember any type of infection—bacterial, viral, or fungal—can lead to sepsis. The ones listed below are the most common causes.*
2	Pneumonia
3	Abdominal infection
4	Kidney infection
5	Bloodstream infection (bacteremia)

Sepsis Risk Factors

1	Patients who are very young or very old
2	Patients who have a compromised immune system
3	Patients who are already very sick such as ICU patients
4	Patients with wounds or injuries such as burns
5	Have invasive devices such as intravenous catheters or breathing tubes

Chapter 24

SUBSTANCE ABUSE

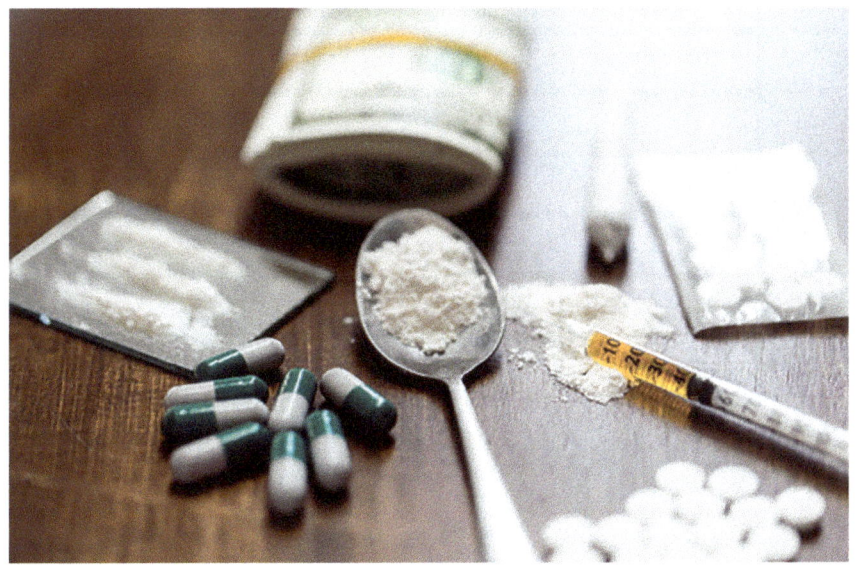

Drugs of Abuse

1	Cocaine
2	Crack
3	Heroin
4	MDMA (ecstasy)
5	Fentanyl
6	Methamphetamine
7	LSD
8	GHB
9	Ketamine
10	PCP
11	Salvia
12	Bath salts
13	Marijuana

Cocaine

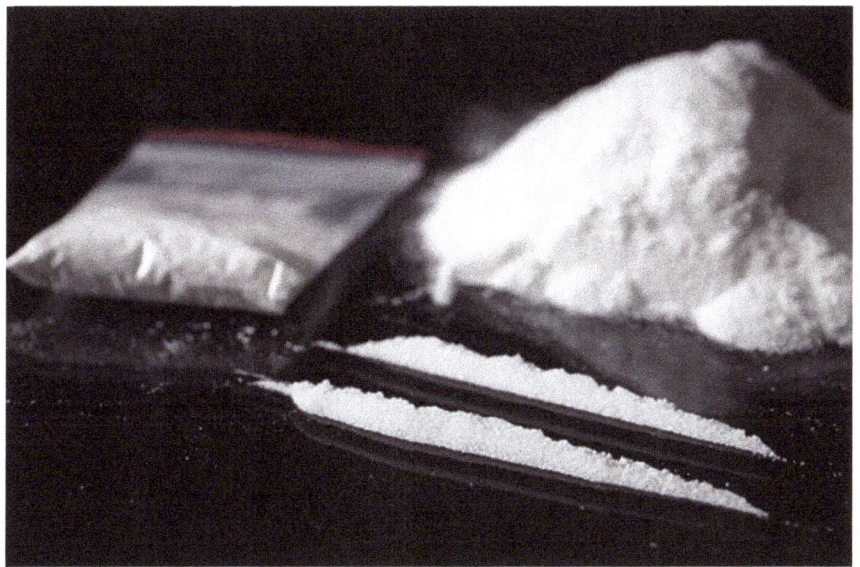

About	Cocaine is a powerfully addictive stimulant drug made from the leaves of the coca plant native to South America. Recreational cocaine use is illegal. As a street drug, cocaine looks like a fine, white, crystal powder. Street dealers often mix it with things like cornstarch, talcum powder, or flour to increase profits. They may also mix it with other drugs such as the stimulant amphetamine or synthetic opioids, including fentanyl.
Street names	• Blow • Coke • Crack • Rock • Snow

How it is used	People snort cocaine powder through the nose, or they rub it into their gums. Others dissolve the powder and inject it into the bloodstream. Some people inject a combination of cocaine and heroin called a speedball. Another popular method of use is to smoke cocaine that has been processed to make a rock crystal (also called "freebase cocaine"). The crystal is heated to produce vapors that are inhaled into the lungs. This form of cocaine is called crack, which refers to the crackling sound of the rock as it is heated. Some people also smoke crack by sprinkling it on marijuana or tobacco and smoke it like a cigarette. People who use cocaine often take it in binges—taking the drug repeatedly within a short time at increasingly higher doses to maintain their high.
Effects on the body	<ul><li>Extreme happiness and energymental alertness</li><li>Hypersensitivity to sight, sound, and touch irritability</li><li>Paranoia—extreme and unreasonable distrust ofothers</li><li>Constricted blood vessels</li><li>Dilated pupils</li><li>Nausea</li><li>Raised body temperature and blood pressure</li><li>Fast or irregular heartbeat</li><li>Tremors and muscle twitches</li><li>Restlessness</li></ul>

Crack Cocaine

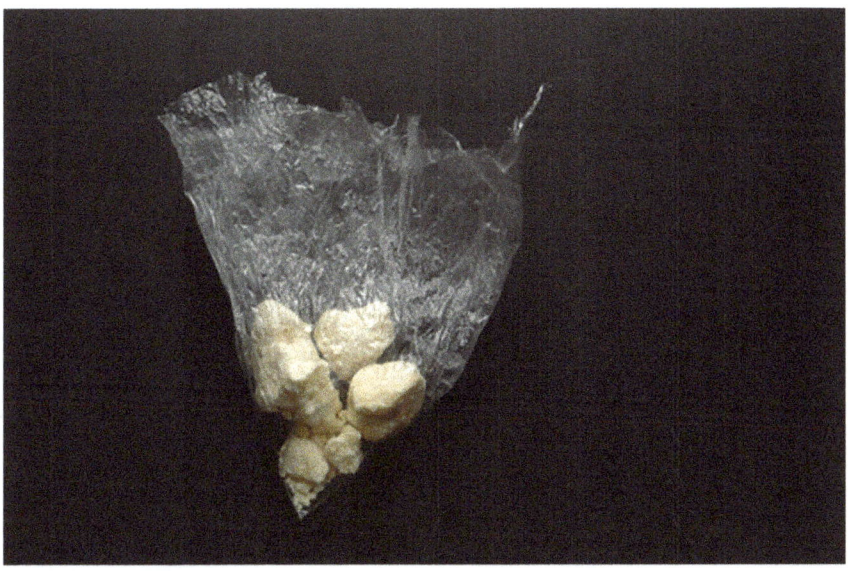

About	Crack cocaine, aka crack, is the freebase form of cocaine. Freebase meaning freeing the cocaine base from the salt form. This makes the cocaine almost 100 percent pure, which leads to a very short intense high period. The effects are felt immediately after use about one to fifteen seconds after use. The highonly lasts about thirty minutes. Because of this, crack cocaine is incredibly addictive to its users.
Street names	• Coke • Snow coke • Hard rock • Candy • Tornado • Gravel • Nuggets • Ice cube • Sugar block

How it is used	Typically smoked
Effects on the body	Short-term effects: - Excessive sweating - Nausea - Pinpoint pupils - Insomnia - Headaches - Decline in sexual function Long-term effects: - Mood changes - Irritability - Restlessness - Depression - Anxiety - Paranoia - Hallucinations

Heroin

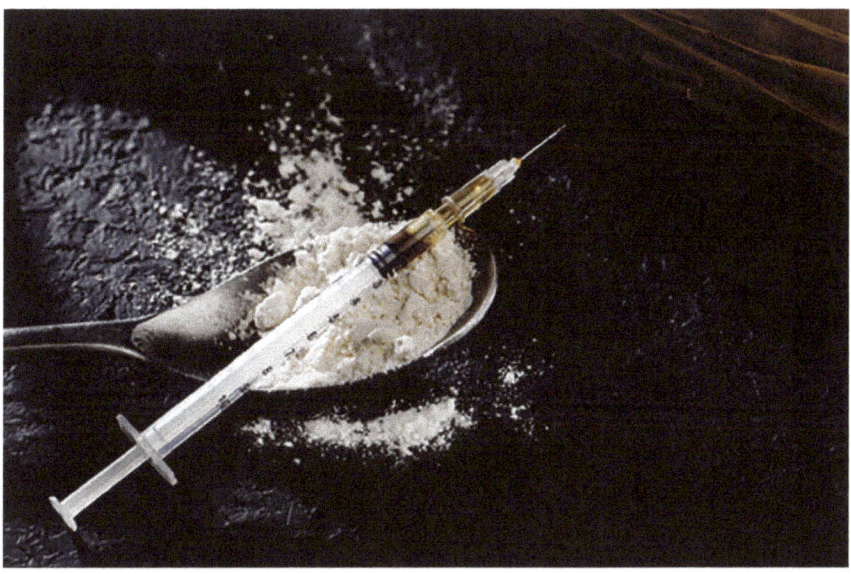

About	Heroin is an opioid drug made from morphine. Heroin can be a white or brown powder or a black sticky substance known as black tar heroin. Because heroin is an opioid, people develop a tolerance to it and then need more of the drug to get the same effect, which typically leads to overdosing.
Street names	<ul><li>Mexican Mud</li><li>Smack</li><li>Dope</li><li>Dragon</li><li>China White</li><li>Scag</li><li>Skunk</li><li>White Horse</li><li>Big H</li></ul>

How it is used	People inject, sniff, snort, or smoke heroin. Some people mix heroin with crack cocaine, a practice called *speedballing*.
Effects on the body	Short-term effects: • Dry mouth • Warm flushing of the skin • Heavy feeling in the arms and legs • Nausea and vomiting • Severe itching • Clouded mental functioning • Back-and-forth state of being conscious and unconscious Long-term effects: • Insomnia • Collapsed veins for people who inject the drug • Damaged tissue inside the nose for people who sniff or snort it • Infection of the heart lining and valves • Abscesses (swollen tissue filled with pus) • Constipation and stomach cramping • Liver and kidney disease • Lung complications, including pneumoniasexual dysfunction for men • Irregular menstrual cycles for women

MDMA (Ecstasy)

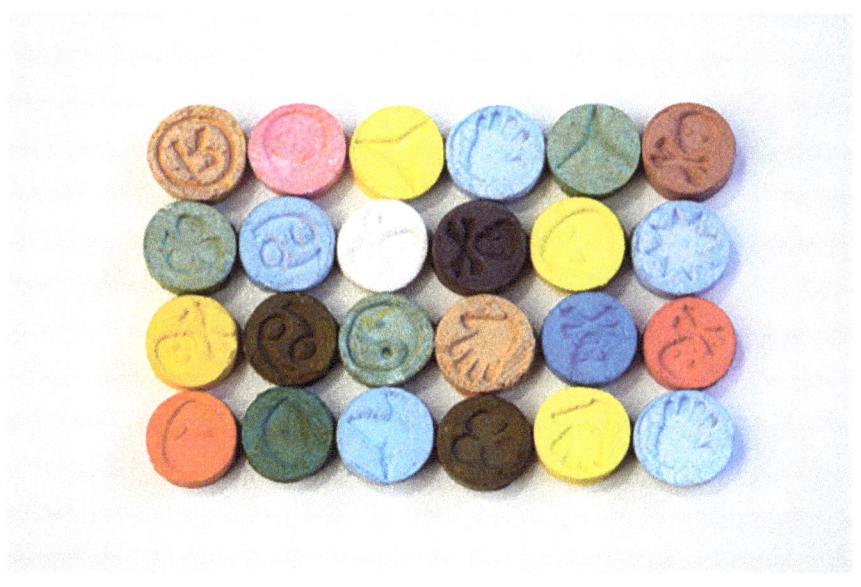

About	The *3,4-methylenedioxymethamphetamine (MDMA)* is a synthetic drug that alters mood and perception (awareness of surrounding objects and conditions). It is chemically similar to both stimulants and hallucinogens, producing feelings of increased energy, pleasure, emotional warmth, and distorted sensory and time perception. MDMA was initially popular in the nightclub scene and at all-night dance parties ("raves"), but the drug now affects a broader range of people who more commonly call the drug *ecstasy* or *Molly*. *MDMA's effects last about three to six hours and typically take about forty-five minutes to kick in after use.* Although many users take a second dose as the effects of the first dose begin to fade.

Street names	- Molly - E, X, XTC - Skittles - Scooby snacks - Thizz - Happy pill - Love drug - Malcolm X - Disco biscuits
How it's used	People who use MDMA usually take it as a capsule or tablet, though some swallow it in liquid form or snort the powder. The popular nickname Molly (slang for "molecular") often refers to the supposedly "pure" crystalline powder form of MDMA, usually sold in capsules.
Effects on the body	MDMA increases the activity of three brain chemicals: - *Dopamine*—produces increased energy/activity and acts in the reward system to reinforce behaviors. - *Norepinephrine*—increases heart rate and blood pressure, which are particularly risky for people with heart and blood vessel problems. - *Serotonin*—affects mood, appetite, sleep, and other functions. It also triggers hormones that affect sexual arousal and trust. The release of large amounts of serotonin likely causes the emotional closeness, elevated mood, and empathy felt by those who use MDMA.

Fentanyl

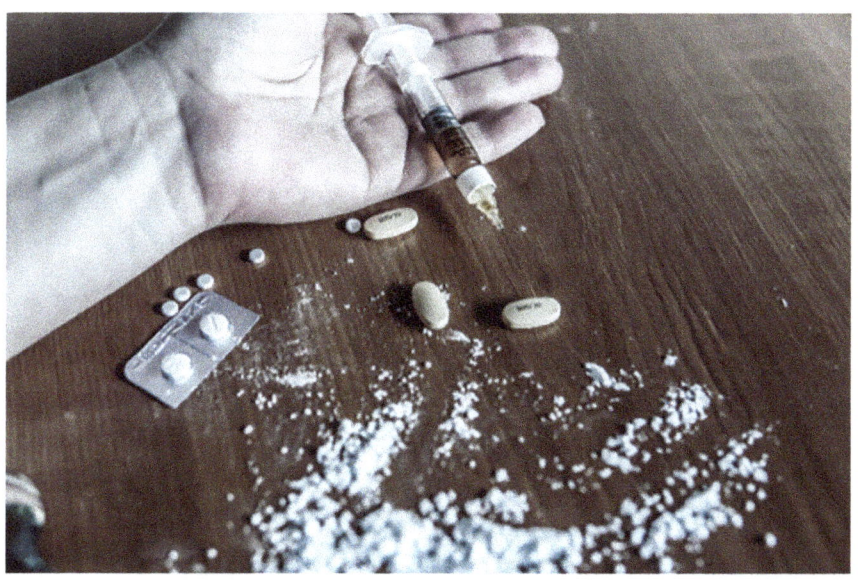

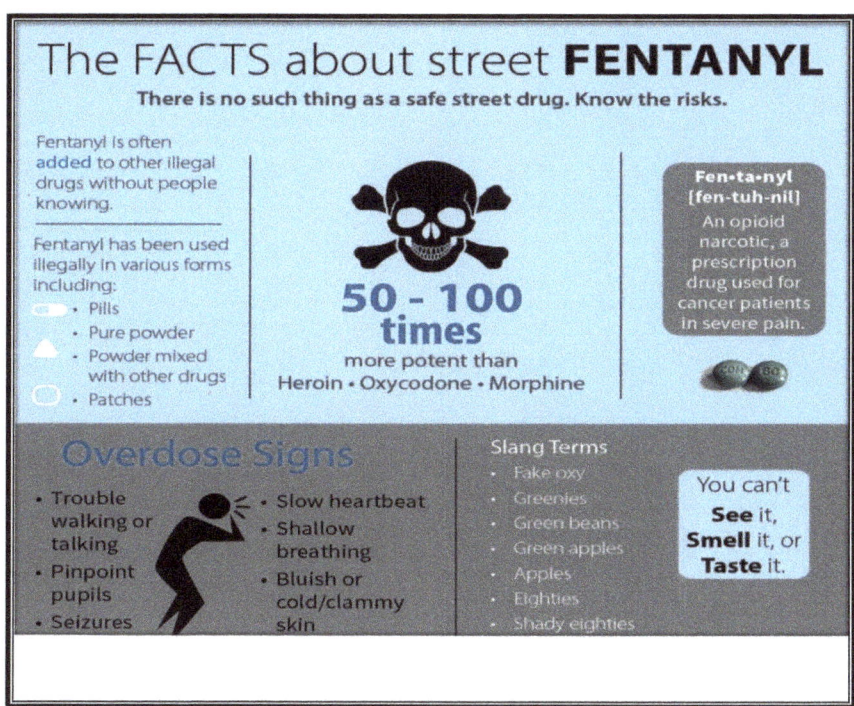

About	Fentanyl was originally invented to relieve pain and is often injected in patients prior to surgical procedures due to its fast-acting, pain-relieving capabilities. Since then, fentanyl has made its way onto the streets and is frequently abused. Fentanyl is now commonly appearing in heroin, cocaine, and marijuana, and overdoses are becoming increasingly more common on the streets.
Street names	<ul><li>Apache</li><li>Dance fever</li><li>Kackpot</li><li>TNT</li><li>Goodfella</li><li>Tango and cash (when mixed with heroin)</li></ul>
How it's used	Fentanyl can be ingested orally or injected.
Effects on the body	<ul><li>Euphoria</li><li>Drowsiness</li><li>Relaxation</li><li>Difficulty concentrating</li><li>Constricted pupils</li><li>Slowed breathing</li><li>Nausea</li><li>Vomiting</li><li>Constipation</li><li>Loss of appetite</li><li>Sweating</li><li>Overdose</li></ul>

Methamphetamine

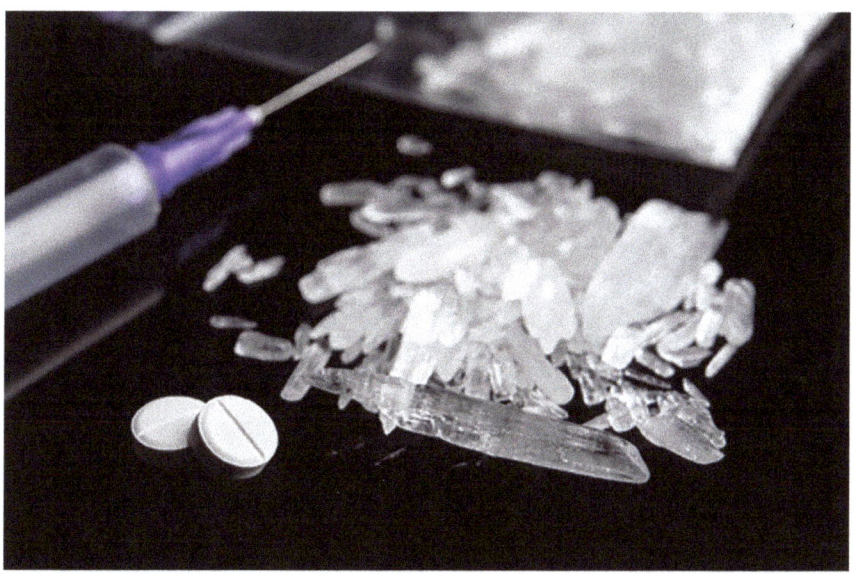

About	Methamphetamine is a stimulant drug usually used as a white, bitter-tasting powder or a pill. Crystal methamphetamine is a form of the drug that looks like glass fragments or shiny, bluish-white rocks.
Street names	• Chalk • Crank • Crystal • Ice • Meth • Speed
How it is used	• Inhaling/smoking • Swallowing (pill) • Snorting • Injecting the powder that has been dissolved in water/alcohol

Effects on the body	Methamphetamine increases the amount of the natural chemical dopamine in the brain. Dopamine is involved in body movement, motivation, and reinforcement of rewarding behaviors. *The drug's ability to rapidly release high levels of dopamine in reward areas of the brain strongly reinforces drug-taking behavior, making the user want to repeat the experience.* Short-term effects: • Increased wakefulness and physical activity decreased appetite • Faster breathing • Rapid and/or irregular heartbeat • Increased blood pressure and body temperature Long-term effects • Extreme weight loss • Severe dental problems ("meth mouth") • Intense itching, leading to skin sores from scratching anxiety • Confusion sleeping problems violent behavior • Paranoia—extreme and unreasonable distrust of other's hallucinations • Sensations and images that seem real though they are not

LSD

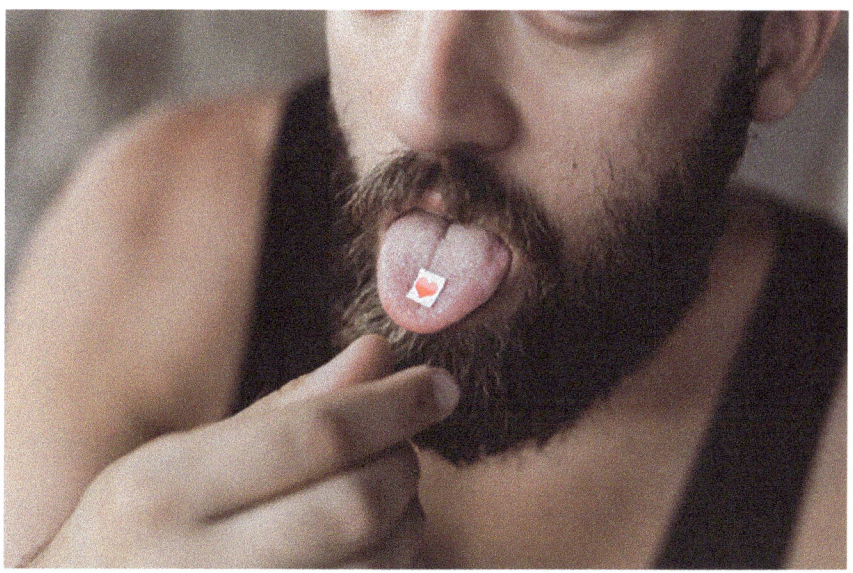

| About | Lysergic acid diethylamide (LSD) is a common recreational drug. It is also commonly known as acid.
LSD is a psychedelic. Psychedelics are drugs that can induce an altered state, perhaps best described as a dreamlike state, for some number of minutes or hours, depending on the specific psychedelic.
LSD generally lasts eight to thirteen hours but expect it to work up to sixteen to eighteen hours.
LSD is also relatively safe if taken properly. |
|---|---|

Street names	Acid California Sunshine Loony Toons Dots Blotter Yellow sunshine Superman
How it is used	LSD is usually consumed on small pieces of paper called blotter.
Effects on the body	Acid feels like "seeing the world for the first time," with stimulated and profound seeming thoughts, and sort of a dreamlike feeling. Hallucinations also exist, though it would be more accurate to think of them as visual distortions (i.e., seeing extra patterns in the grass, a photo of a waterfall might look like the water is moving when it's actually not), but don't think of it as you'll be seeing green leprechauns that will talk to you. Some effects are: • Hallucination • Anxiety • Paranoid thinking • Discomfort • May increase blood pressure • Joy and intense happiness

GHB

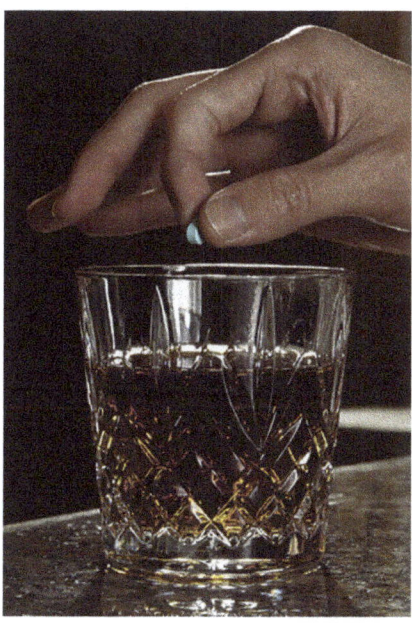

About	GHB or gamma-hydroxybutyrate (C4H8O3) is a central nervous system (CNS) depressant that is commonly referred to as a "club drug" or "date rape" drug. GHB is abused by teens and young adults at bars, parties, clubs, and "raves" (all-night dance parties) and is often placed in alcoholic beverages.
Street names	<ul><li>Soap</li><li>Liquid XTC</li><li>Candy</li><li>Raver</li><li>Everclear cherry meth</li><li>Fantasy</li><li>G-riffic</li></ul>

How it's used	*GHB is available as an odorless, colorless drug that may be combined with alcohol and given to unsuspecting victims prior to sexual assaults.* It may have a soapy or salty taste. Use for sexual assault has resulted in GHB being known as a "date rape" drug. Victims become incapacitated due to the sedative effects of GHB, and they are unable to resist sexual assault. GHB may also induce amnesia in its victim. Common user groups include high school and college students and rave party attendees who use GHB for its intoxicating effects.
Effects on the Body	<ul><li>Sweating</li><li>Loss of consciousness</li><li>Nausea</li><li>Auditory and visual hallucinations</li><li>Headaches</li><li>Vomiting</li><li>Exhaustion</li><li>Sluggishness</li><li>Amnesia</li><li>Confusion</li><li>Clumsiness</li></ul>

Ketamine

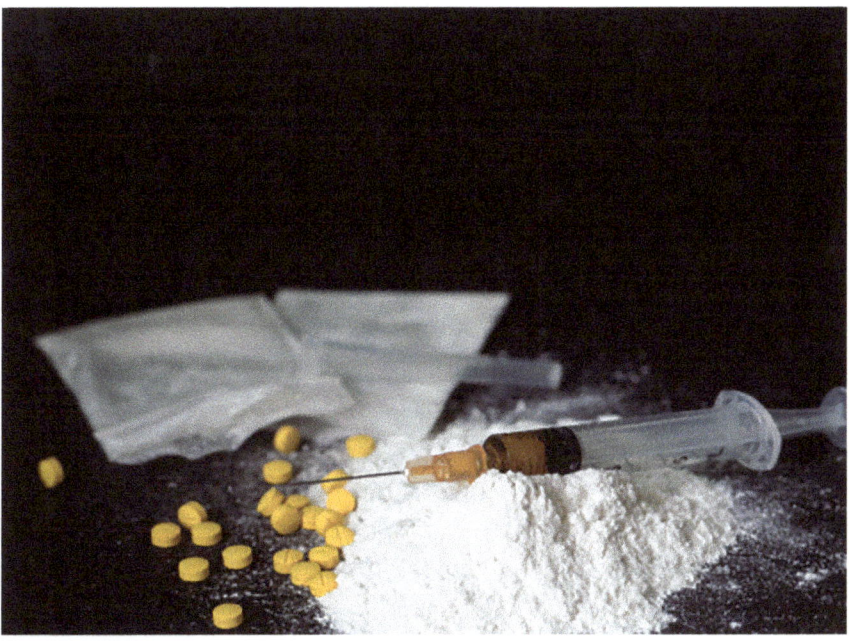

About	*Ketamine is a dissociative anesthetic used in human anesthesia and veterinary medicine.* Dissociative drugs are hallucinogens that cause a person to feel detached from reality. Much of the ketamine sold on the street has been diverted from veterinarians' offices. Ketamine's chemical structure and mechanism of action are like those of PCP.
Street names	- Special K - Super acid - Kit Kat - Purple - Vitamin K

How it's used	Ketamine is snorted or swallowed. Ketamine is odorless and tasteless, so it can be added to beverages without being detected, and it induces amnesia. Ketamine is also considered to be a "date rape" drug because it has been used to commit sexual assaults due to its ability to sedate and incapacitate unsuspecting victims, preventing them from resisting sexual assault.
Effects on the body	• Impaired attention, learning ability, and memory • Delirium • Amnesia • Impaired motor function • High blood pressure • Depression

PCP (Angel Dust)

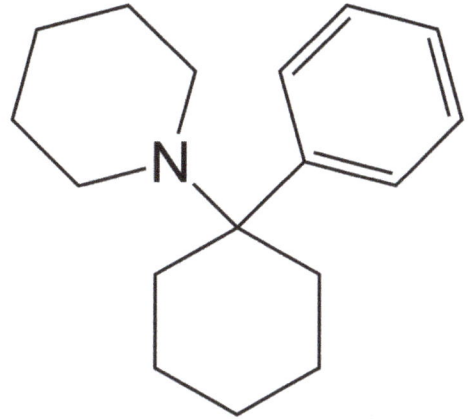

About	*Phencyclidine (PCP) is a mind-altering drug that may lead to hallucinations (a profound distortion in a person's perception of reality).* It is considered a dissociative drug, leading to a distortion of sights, colors, sounds, self, and one's environment. PCP was developed in the 1950s as an intravenous anesthetic, but due to the serious neurotoxic side effects, its development for human medical use was discontinued. *In its purest form, PCP is a white crystalline powder that readily dissolves in water or alcohol* and has a distinctive bitter chemical taste. On the illicit drug market, PCP contains several contaminants causing the color to range from a light to darker brown with a powdery to a gummy mass consistency.

Street names	- Angel dust - Ozone - Rocket fuel - Love boat - Embalming fluid - Hog - Superweed - Wack - Wet (a marijuana joint dipped in PCP)
How it's used	PCP is available in a variety of tablets, capsules, and colored powders, which are either smoked, taken orally, or by the intranasal route ("snorted"). Smoking is the most common route when used recreationally. The liquid form of PCP is actually PCP base, often dissolved in either a highly flammable solvent. For smoking, PCP is typically sprayed onto leafy materials such as mint, parsley, oregano, or marijuana. PCP may also be injected. *The effects of PCP can last for four to six hours.*
Effects on the body	- Feeling of detachment - Numbness to extremities - Slurred speech - Loss of coordination - Rapid involuntary eye movements - Auditory hallucinations - Image distortion - Amnesia - Anxiety - Paranoia - Psychosis

Physiological effects of high doses:

- Slight increase in breathing rate
- Rise in blood pressure and pulse rate
- Shallow respiration
- Flushing and profuse sweating occurs

Physiological effects of high doses of PCP include:

- A drop in blood pressure, pulse rate, and respiration
- Nausea
- Vomiting
- Blurred vision
- Flicking up and down of the eyes
- Drooling
- Loss of balance and dizziness
- Violence
- Suicide

Salvia

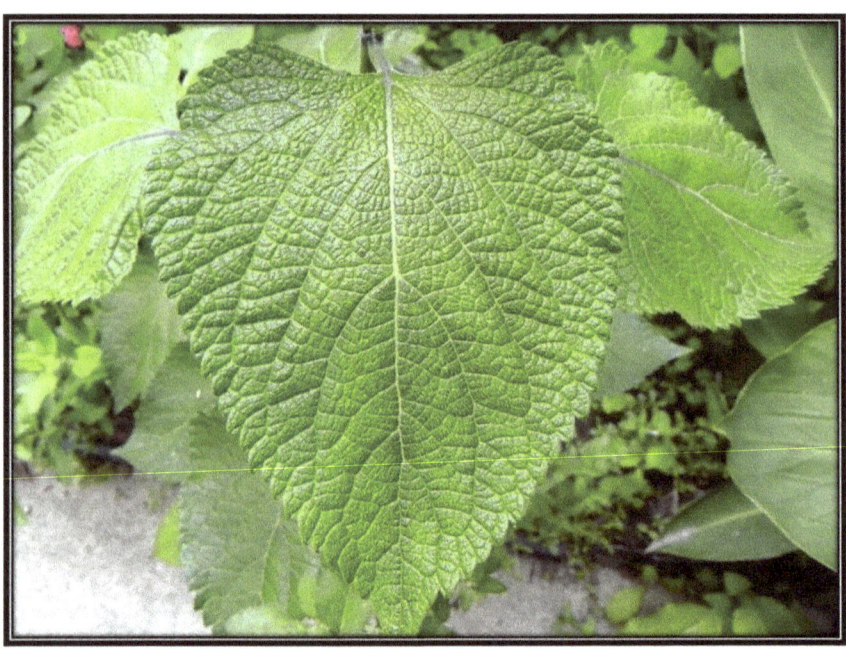

About	*Salvia (Salvia divinorum)* is a plant of the mint family common in southern Mexico and Central and South America. *Salvia is a dissociative hallucinogenic drug.* Its main active ingredient (salvinorin A) attaches to elements of the kappa opioid receptors, which regulate human perception. *The effects of salvia are quick to reach their peak after five to twenty-five minutes and last for around thirty minutes, depending on the method of ingestion and the quantity used.* Smoking salvia produces effects more quickly. While taken orally, it acts slower but with longer effects—around sixty to 120 minutes.

Street names	- Leaves of Mary - The shepherdess - Diviner's Sage - Diviner's mint - Sally-D - Magic mint
How it's used	- Chewing, also known as quidding - Smoking - Vaporizing
Effects on the body	Salvia use has powerful psychological effects: - Hallucinations - Changes in vision, mood, and sensations - Extreme emotional swings - Detachment from self, reality, and surroundings, causing loss of perception between what's real and what's not People who used salvia also reported the following effects: - Visual alterations - Uncontrollable laughter - Extreme confusion - Loss of sense of individual awareness - Hallucinations of flying, twisting, spinning - Appearances of travel in time and space - Intensified sensory experiences like unifying with objects out of body experiences

Some common adverse physical side-effects of salvia are:

- Nausea,
- Loss of physical coordination
- Slurred speech
- Irregular heart rate
- Increased breathing rate

Bath Salts

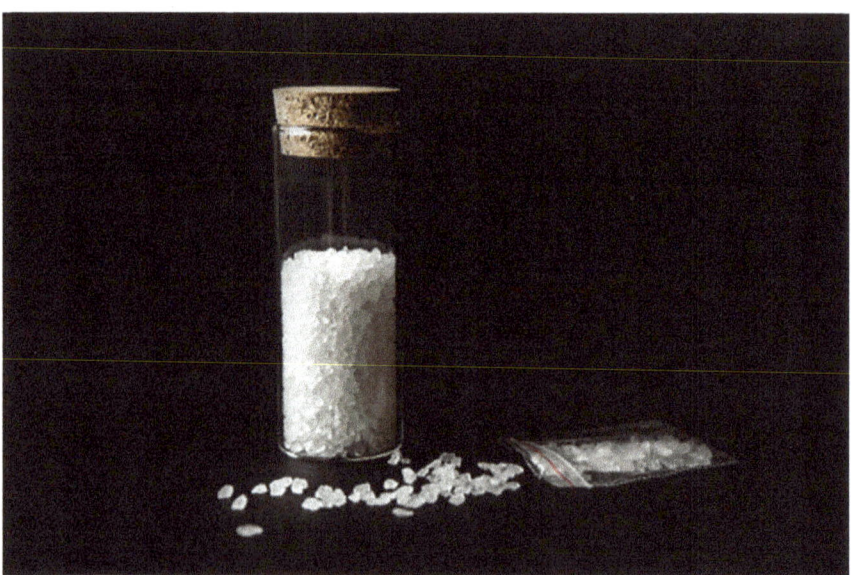

About

Synthetic cathinones, more commonly known as "bath salts," are human-made stimulants chemically related to cathinone, a substance found in the khat plant. Khat is a shrub grown in East Africa and southern Arabia where some people chew its leaves for their mild stimulant effects.

	Human-made versions of cathinone can be much stronger than the natural product and, in some cases, very dangerous.
Street names	• Cloud 9 • Vanilla sky • White lightning • Bloom • Scarface • Bliss • Drone • Energy-1 • Meow-Meow
How it's used	• Swallow • Snort • Smoke • Inject
Effects on the body	• Paranoia • Hallucinations • Increased friendliness • Increased sex drive • Panic attacks • Excited delirium—extreme agitation and violent behavior

Marijuana

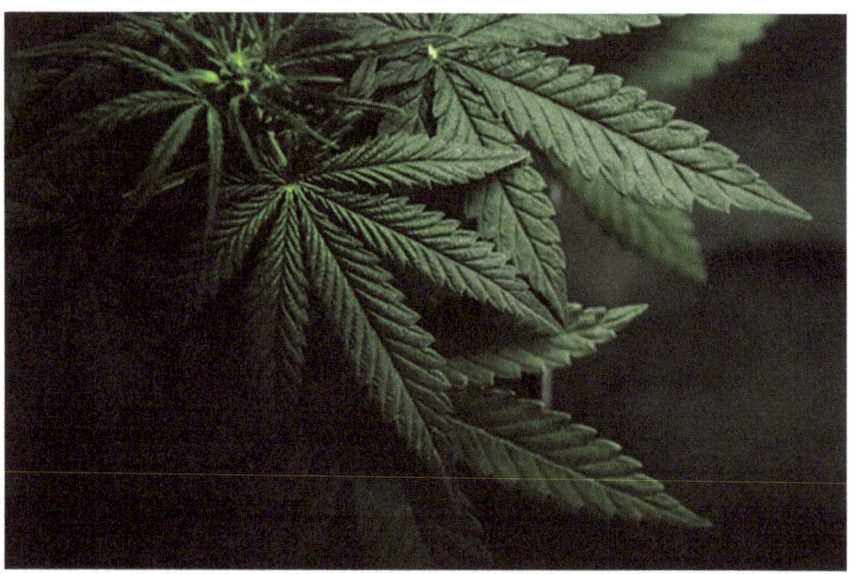

About	Marijuana refers to the dried leaves, flowers, stems, and seeds from the *Cannabis sativa* or *Cannabis indica* plant. The plant contains the mind-altering chemical THC and other similar compounds. Marijuana is the most commonly used drug in the United States.
Street names	• Weed • Pot • Reefer • Grass • Dope • Ganja • Mary Jane • Hash • Herb • Aunt Mary

How it is used	- Smoke
- Ingest

People smoke marijuana in hand-rolled cigarettes (joints) or in pipes or water pipes (bongs). They also smoke it in blunts—emptied cigars that have been partly or completely refilled with marijuana. To avoid inhaling smoke, some people use vaporizers. These devices pull the active ingredients (including THC) from the marijuana and collect their vapor in a storage unit. A person then inhales the vapor, not the smoke. Some vaporizers use a liquid marijuana extract.

People can mix marijuana in food (edibles), such as brownies, cookies, or candy or brew it as a tea. A newly popular method of use is smoking or eating different forms of THC-rich resins. |
| Effects on the body | Short-term effects:

- Altered senses (for example, seeing brighter colors)
- Altered sense of time
- Changes in mood
- Impaired body movement
- Difficulty with thinking and problem-solving
- Impaired memory
- Hallucinations (when taken in high doses)
- Delusions (when taken in high doses)
- Psychosis (when taken in high doses) |

Long-term effects:

Marijuana also affects brain development. When people begin using marijuana as teenagers, the drug may impair thinking, memory, and learning functions and affect how the brain builds connections between the areas necessary for these functions. Researchers are still studying how long marijuana's effects last and whether some changes may be permanent.

Chapter 25

SYNCOPE/FALLS

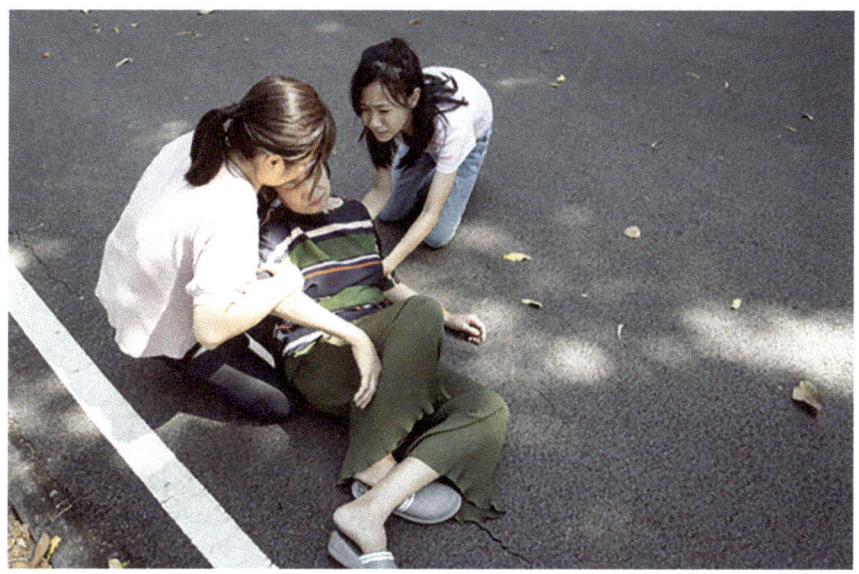

Syncope *(Greek – to interrupt)*

- **Syncope** is the sudden transient loss of consciousness and postural tone with spontaneous recovery.
- **Loss of consciousness** occurs within 10 seconds of hypoperfusion of the reticular activating system in the mid brain

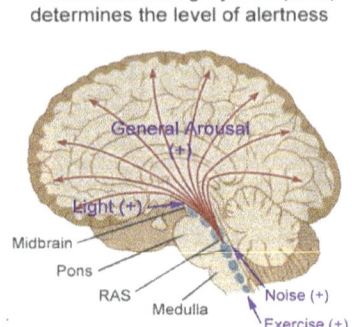

Reticular Activating System (RAS) determines the level of alertness

Questions to Ask

1	Can the patient recall what happened prior to the event? What is their GCS score and A&O status?
2	How did the patient fall? Was it mechanical? Did the patient have a medical complaint before falling such as feeling dizzy or lightheaded?
3	What was the height the patient fell from? Does it meet trauma criteria?
3	What surface did they fall onto? Was it carpet, concrete, tile, grass?

3	Did the patient hit their head? Palpate and check for trauma.
4	Any loss of consciousness?
5	Any head, neck, or midline back pain?
6	Any numbness or tingling to extremities? Check CSM.
7	Is the patient taking any blood thinners (see list below)?
8	Perform a head-to-toe assessment and clear C spine if appropriate.
9	Does the patient have any medical complaints? Any chest pain, shortness of breath, nausea, vomiting, diarrhea, headache, dizziness, blurred vision, recent illnesses, fever, body aches, chills, weakness, or any recent drug or alcohol use?
10	Does the patient have any pain anywhere or injuries that need to be treated?

Causes of Syncope

1	Hypotension/dilated blood vessels
2	Cardiac arrhythmias (irregular heartbeat)
3	Abrupt changes in posture, such as standing up too quickly, which can cause blood to pool in the feet or legs (*check orthostatic vital signs*)
4	Standing for long periods of time
5	Extreme pain or fear
6	Extreme stress

7	Pregnancy
8	Dehydration
9	Exhaustion
10	Hypoglycemia

Syncopal Episodes Warning Signs and Symptoms

1	Nausea
2	Slurred speech
3	Weak pulse
4	Sudden clammy sweat
5	Feeling as if sounds are suddenly very far away and ringing in the ears
6	Disturbances to your vision
7	Pale skin
8	Vertigo
9	Shakiness
10	Headache
11	Rapid heartbeat
12	Body weakness

Treatment Syncope

1	Vital signs (orthostatic)
2	Blood sugar
3	Stroke assessment
4	12-lead EKG
5	IV
6	Normal saline if appropriate

How to Check Orthostatic Vital Signs

Orthostatic vital signs may be indicated to evaluate patients who are at risk for hypovolemia (vomiting, diarrhea, bleeding), have had syncope or near syncope (dizziness, fainting), or are at risk for falls. A significant change in vital signs with a change in position also signals increased risk for falls.

Orthostatic hypotension is defined as a decrease in systolic blood pressure of 20 mm Hg or a decrease in diastolic blood pressure of 10 mmHg within three minutes of standing when compared with blood pressure from the sitting or supine position.

Obtain a BP with the patient lying down, sitting, then standing. Check for a change in HR and BP for positive Orthostatics.

Chapter 26

ALLERGIC REACTION

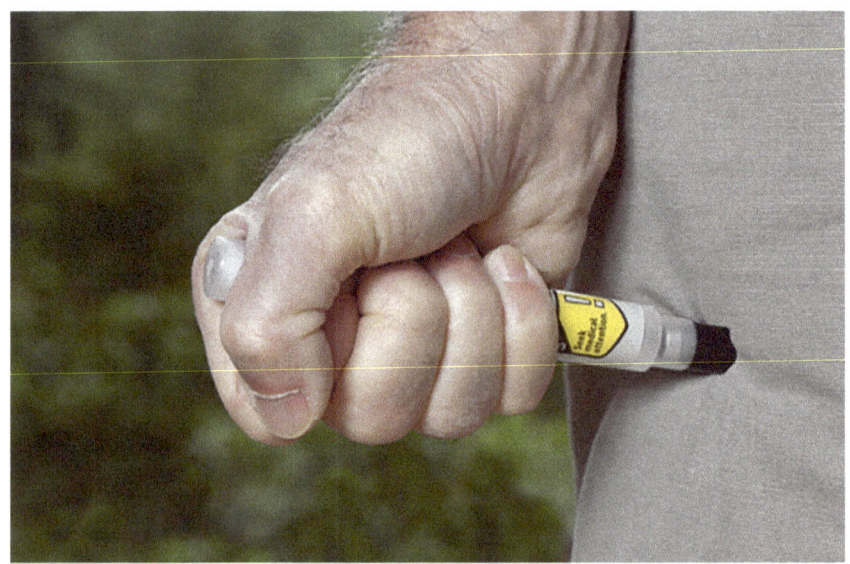

What is an allergic reaction?	*An allergy occurs when the body's immune system sees a substance as harmful and overreacts to it. When a person who is allergic to a particular allergen comes into contact with it, an allergic reaction occurs.* This begins when the allergen (for example, pollen) enters the body, triggering an antibody response. The antibodies attach themselves to special cells called mast cells. When the pollen comes into contact with the antibodies, the mast cells respond by releasing certain substances, one of which is called histamine. When the release of histamine is due to an allergen, the resulting swelling and inflammation are extremely irritating and uncomfortable.
Allergen types	• Drugs (medicine) • Food • Insects that sting (bee, wasp, fire ant); bite (mosquito, tick); or are household pests (cockroach and dust mite) • Latex • Mold • Pollen • Pet (dog or cat urine, saliva, and dander)

How an Allergy is Diagnosed

The patient's doctor should perform some of the following tests. A good question you can ask your patient is if they have gotten any of these tests performed and already know what they are allergic to.

Anaphylaxis

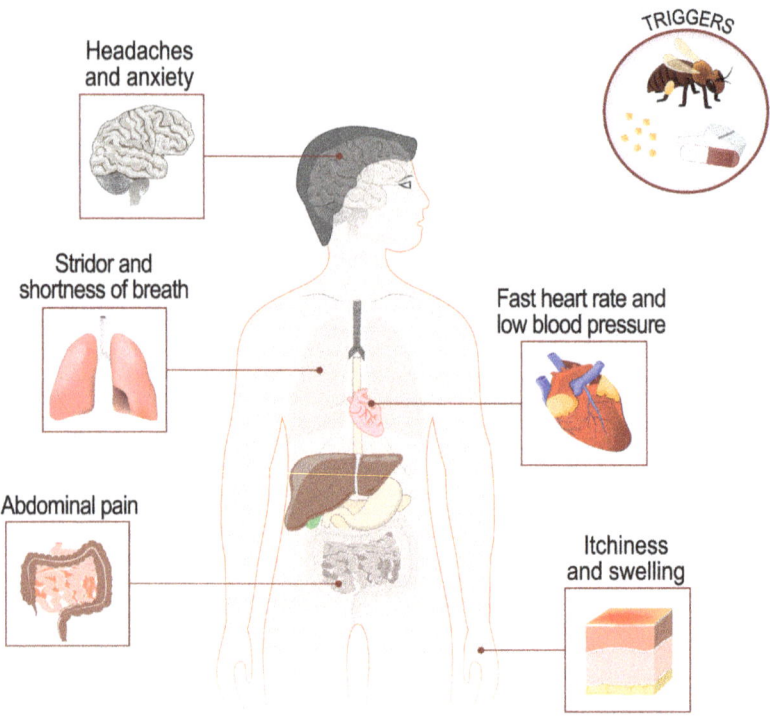

Skin tests	A skin test involves applying a small amount of a suspected allergen to the skin and watching for a reaction. The substance may be taped to the skin (patch test), applied via a small prick to the skin (skin prick test), or injected just under the skin (intradermal test). A skin test is most valuable for diagnosing the following: • Food allergy • Mold, pollen, and animal dander allergy

	- Penicillin allergy - Venom allergy (mosquito bite or bee sting) - Allergic contact dermatitis (a rash you get from touching a substance)
Blood tests	A blood test for an allergy checks your blood for antibodies against a possible allergen. An antibody is a protein your body produces to fight harmful substances. Blood tests are an option when skin testing is not helpful or possible.
Challenge (elimination-type) test	Challenge testing is useful in diagnosing food allergies. It involves removing a food from your diet for several weeks and watching for symptoms when you eat the food again.

Hives (Urticaria)

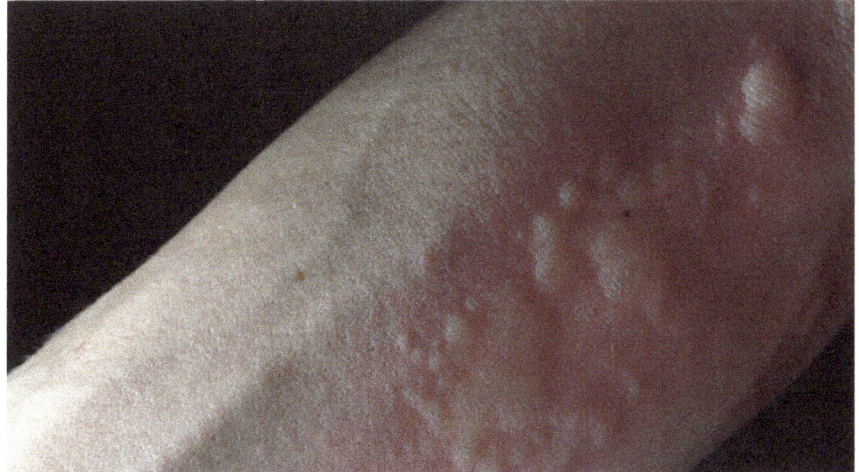

Chapter 27

DEATH IN THE FIELD

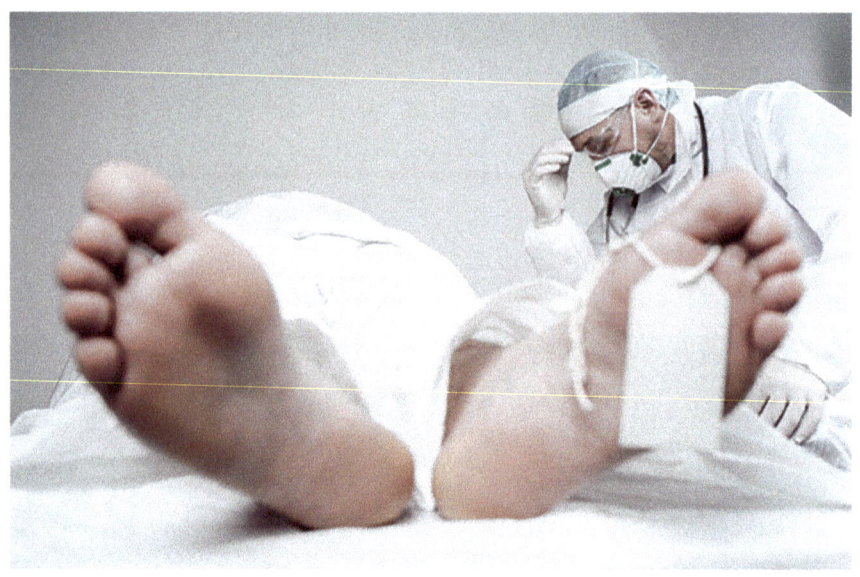

Information to Obtain Prior to Calling the Medical Examiner

1	Patient's name
2	Home address with cross street
3	What kind of death was it? Suicide, natural causes, etc.?
4	Anything lying around such as empty pill bottles, bottles of alcohol, etc.?
5	Is there a next of kin or any family members around?
6	Were the police notified already? If not, request for them.
7	*Make sure not to touch anything because it is now a crime scene.* (Make sure nobody else touches anything.)

Make sure to follow your own county's death in the field policy. Death in the field policy in San Francisco states the following:

Policy

A. A patient may be determined dead without **b**ase **h**ospital contact when one of the following conditions exist (per SFEMSA policy 4050, effective date January 30, 2017):

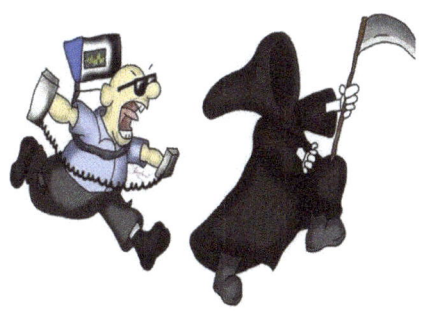

Obvious deaths	• Decapitation • Total incineration • Decomposition • Separation from the body of either the brain, liver, or heart • Rigor mortis (Note: must apply EKG leads and confirm asystole in two leads)
Medical indications	Unwitnessed arrest with a reasonable suspicion of downtime of fifteen minutes or greater *and* the patient is pulseless and apneic (no shock indicated on AED for BLS or asystole in two leads for ALS) *and* no evidence of hypothermia, drug ingestion, or poisoning. Patient has had at least forty minutes of ALS intervention, initial resuscitation efforts have been unsuccessful, and treatment protocols have been exhausted. Patient intubated or supraglottic airway inserted and end-tidal CO_2 monitor shows good waveform (for placement confirmation) and persistent low ETCO2 reading (less than 5 mmHg).
Medical directives	Presence of a valid prehospital do not resuscitate (DNR) or physician orders for life-sustaining treatment (POLST) form and medallion/bracelet form (see Policy 4051 Do Not Resuscitate & Physician Orders for Life-Sustaining Treatment).
Trauma	MCI incident where triage principles preclude initiation of CPR. Blunt, penetrating, or profound multisystem trauma with wide complex PEA < 40 or asystole.

Environmental	Drowning victims where it is reasonably determined that submersion has been thirty minutes or greater.

If CPR was initiated by non-EMS personnel for the above-mentioned conditions listed in 2.A, 1–5, *discontinue CPR.*

The base hospital physician must be contacted to determine death in the field in the following situations:

1. CPR is started on a patient with *no* valid DNR/POLST form and the spouse, immediate family member(s), or guardian who are present disagree on the patient's last wishes for CPR.
2. Any situation in which the paramedic's response warrants clarification or direction.

Chapter 28

SHOCK

The Rapid Progression of Shock

Compensated shock	Decompensated shock	Irreversible shock
• Pulse rate increases • Respirations increase • Weak pulse • Cool, clammy skin • Anxious, restless, combative • Thirsty, weak	• Very weak or absent pulses • Severe drop in blood pressure • Altered mental status or unconsciousness • Slow breathing to apnea	• Cell death • Organ system failure • Washout • Hemorrhaging all over • Patient dies
Stage I and II hemorrhages 500-1250ml blood loss 5-25% blood volume lost	**Stage III and IV hemorrhages** 1250-1750+ ml blood loss 25-35%+ blood volume lost	**Stage IV hemorrhage** 1750+ ml blood loss 35%+ blood volume lost
THIS IS WHERE YOU NEED TO WORK YOUR MAGIC. Stop the bleeding. Oxygenation. Give fluids. Keep the patient warm. Get them to definitive care.	WORK VERY FAST. You MAY be able to get the patient back, but you need to work very fast. Praying helps.	STICK A FORK IN HIM. HE'S DONE.

Types of Shock

Class of haemorrhagic shock				
	I	II	III	IV
Blood loss (mL)	Up to 750	750–1500	1500–2000	> 2000
Blood loss (% blood volume)	Up to 15	15–30	30–40	> 40
Pulse rate (per minute)	< 100	100–120	120–140	> 140
Blood pressure	Normal	Normal	Decreased	Decreased
Pulse pressure (mm Hg)	Normal or increased	Decreased	Decreased	Decreased
Respiratory rate (per minute)	14–20	20–30	30–40	> 35
Urine output (mL/hour)	> 30	20–30	5–15	Negligible
Central nervous system/ mental status	Slightly anxious	Mildly anxious	Anxious, confused	Confused, lethargic

Hypovolemic shock	Decreased blood volume. A type of hypovolemic shock is hemorrhagic shock, which results from blood loss.
	Can also be from the patient losing too much body fluid, which could happen from diarrhea, burns, excessive perspiration, or vomiting.
	Hypovolemic shock is an emergency condition in which severe blood and fluid loss make the heart unable to pump enough blood to the body. This type of shock can cause many organs to stop working. Losing about one-fifth or more of the normal amount of blood in your body causes hypovolemic shock.
Obstructive shock	Something blocks perfusion to the heart. For example, pulmonary embolism, tension pneumothorax, or cardiac tamponade.

Distributive shock	Abnormal blood distribution that leads to inadequate blood reaching the heart. In hypovolemic shock, there is an insufficient volume of blood. This form of relative hypovolemia is the result of dilation of blood vessels. Examples of this form of shock are: • Septic shock • Anaphylactic shock • Neurogenic shock
Neurogenic shock	Nervous system injury leading to vasodilation in the periphery, causing inadequate perfusion to the vital organs. Caused by the sudden loss of the sympathetic nervous system signals to the smooth muscle in vessel walls. Without this constant stimulation, the vessels relax, resulting in a sudden decrease in peripheral vascular resistance and decreased blood pressure. The rarest cause of shock is acute spinal cord injury, leading to neurogenic shock.
Anaphylactic shock	Severe allergic reaction that leads to vasodilation and bronchoconstriction. Caused by allergens that trigger widespread vasodilation and movement of fluid out of the blood into the tissues. This is a serious, potentially life-threatening allergic response that is marked by swelling, lowered blood pressure, and dilated blood vessels. In severe cases, a person will go into shock. If anaphylactic shock is not treated immediately, it can be fatal.

Cardiogenic shock	It is a shock with cardiac origin and an inadequate pumping of the heart. It can be due to heart disease or heart attack. It can also be due to the following: • Acute myocarditis or endocarditis-induced heart failure from drugs/medications (i.e., cocaine, beta-blockers, tricyclic antidepressants); • Trauma-related such as a myocardial contusion; • Metabolic disorders resulting in cardiac arrhythmias such as sustained tachycardia or bradycardia; and • Pulmonary embolism that may also produce cardiogenic shock by impeding blood flow in the pulmonary vessels.
Compensating shock	1. Clammy (pale, cool, and diaphoretic skin) 2. Nausea/vomiting 3. Weak, rapid, thready, or absent distal pulses 4. Shortness of breath 5. Agitation, anxiety, restlessness, feeling of impending doom 6. Altered mental status 7. Delayed capillary refill
Decompensating shock	1. Hypotension 2. Thready or absent pulses 3. Labored or irregular breathing 4. Ashen, mottled, or cyanotic skin 5. Dilated pupils

CHAPTER 29

SCENE MANAGEMENT AND MCI

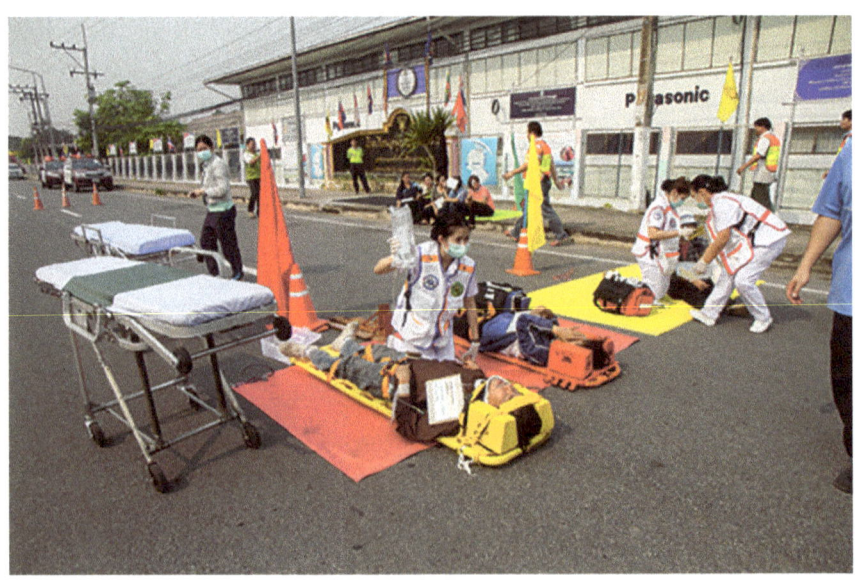

MARK POYER

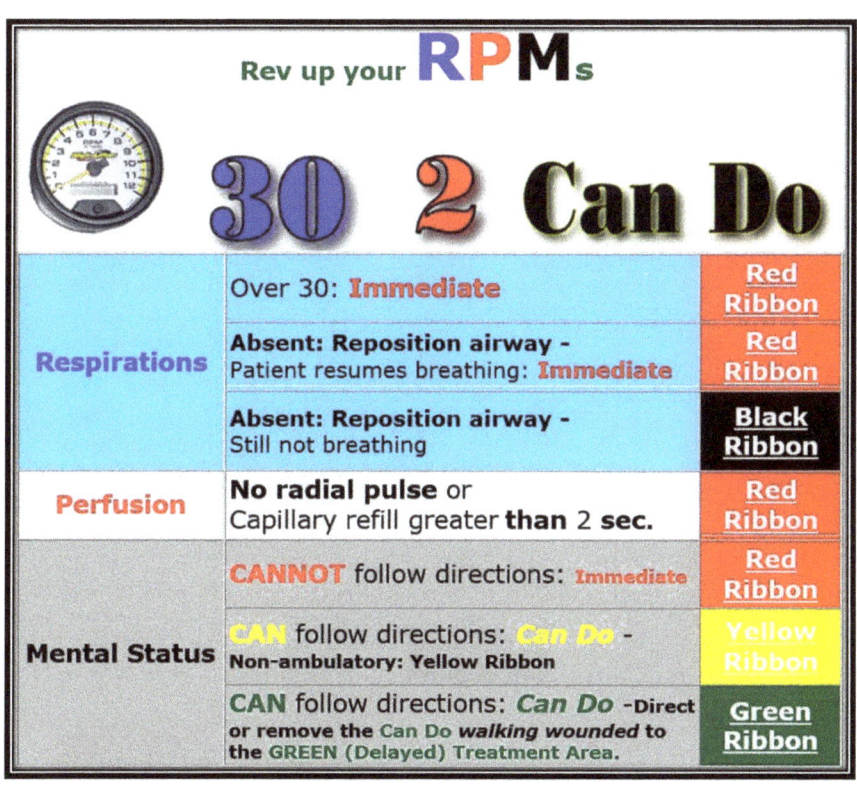

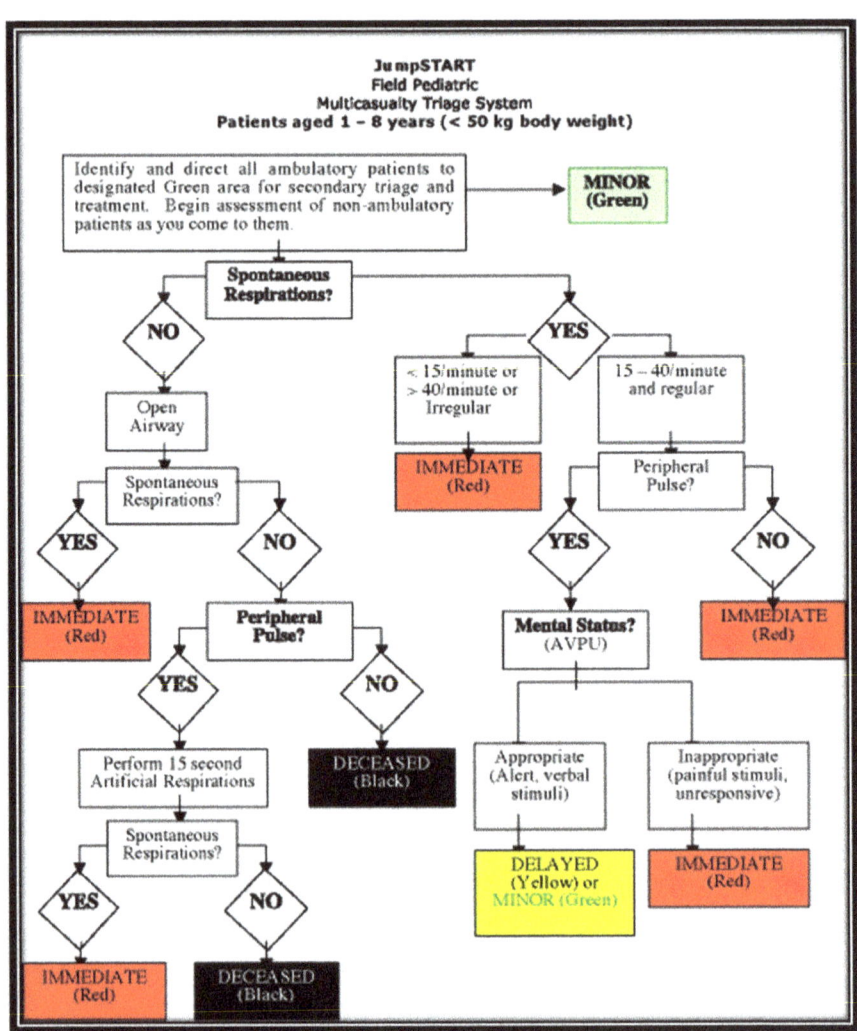

Things to Think About

1	When responding to a call, pay attention to what resources are responding.
2	If you do not need certain resources after you arrive on scene, cut them loose.
3	Look to see if your patient is stable or unstable. Think about if you are going to need an extra set of hands during transport or to help with extrication to get the patient to the ambulance. An example would be needing an extra set of hands with the stair chair.
4	Remember to delegate. Have a game plan when you are running your call. As you're taking the patient to the ambulance, you should already have a game plan established. If you need to free your hands up so you can do a ringdown or start an IV or perform a 12-lead or need someone to monitor the airway then delegate. Free your hands up.

SFEMSA MCI Alert Levels

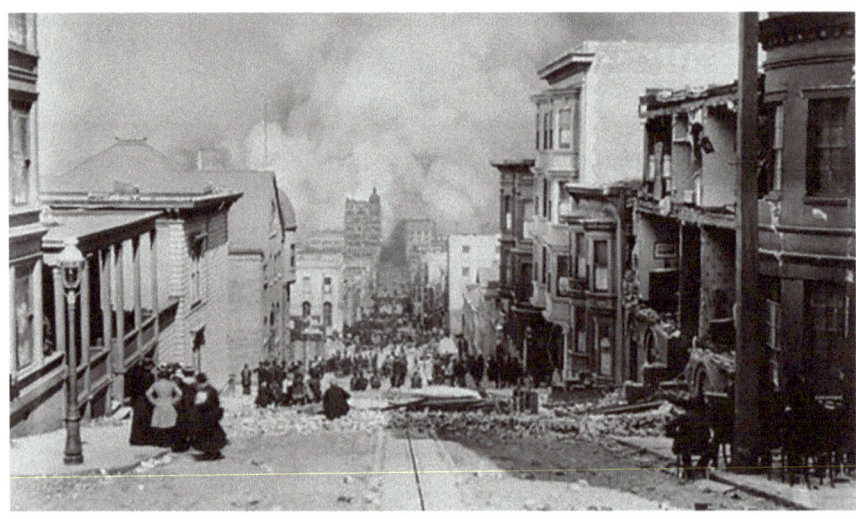

MCI yellow alert	Incident with potential for multiple patients
Level 1 MCI red alert	MCI with 6–50 victims of any triage level
Level 2 MCI red alert	MCI with 51–100 victims of any triage level
Level 3 MCI red alert	MCI with 101 victims of any triage level
Level 4 MCI red alert	Catastrophic disaster (example: earthquake)

MCI

Positions in Order of EMS Response

First ambulance on scene	Paramedic is the medical group supervisor and the EMT is the triage unit leader.
Second ambulance on scene	Paramedic is the treatment unit leader and the EMT is the transport unit leader
Third ambulance on scene	In charge of staging and determining if a medical branch with several medical groups will be established.

SFEMSA Hospitals Can Take the Following During an MCI

SFGH	can take the first ten trauma patients and a total of twenty patients
All other hospitals (twelve patients total)	• Two immediate • Four delayed • Six minors

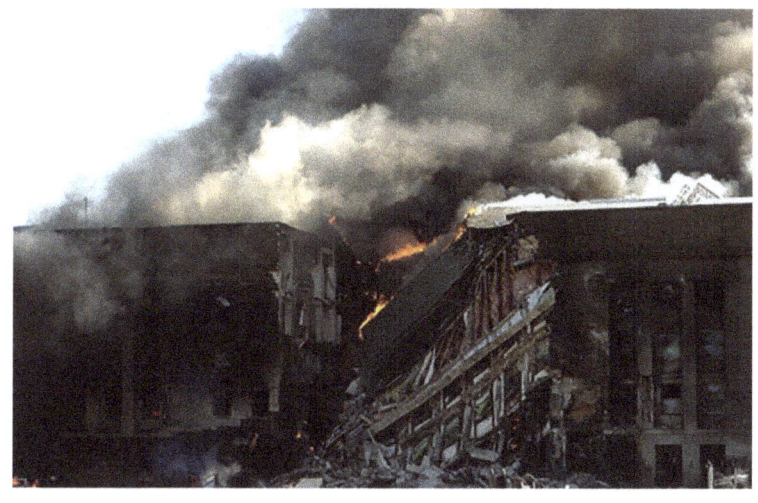

SFEMSA

MCI Incident Command

What to mention on radio channel B15 within the first fifteen minutes:

1	Yellow or red alert and what level
2	Location of incident and name of command
3	Type or nature of the incident
4	Hazards
5	Number of victims
6	Command post and staging locations
7	Initial route of ingress and egress
8	Any special resources if needed

Chapter 30

DIALYSIS

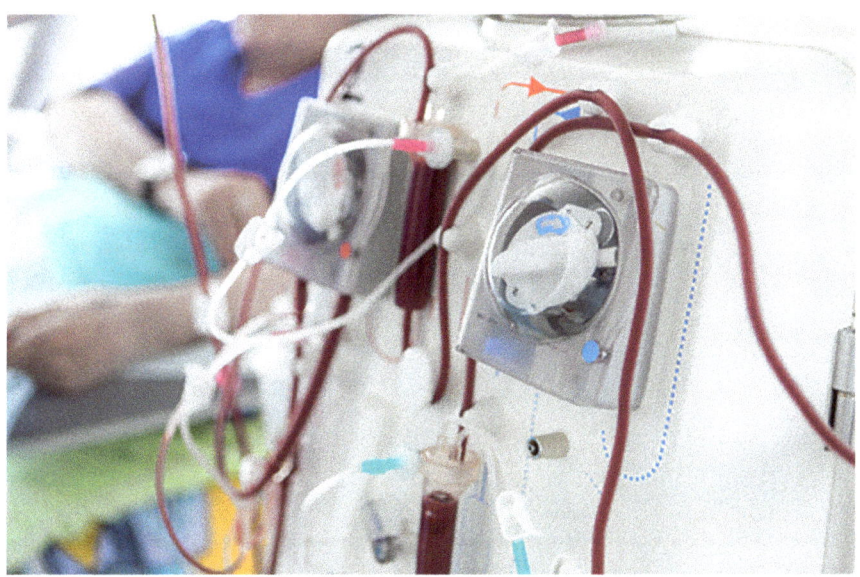

Dialysis Information

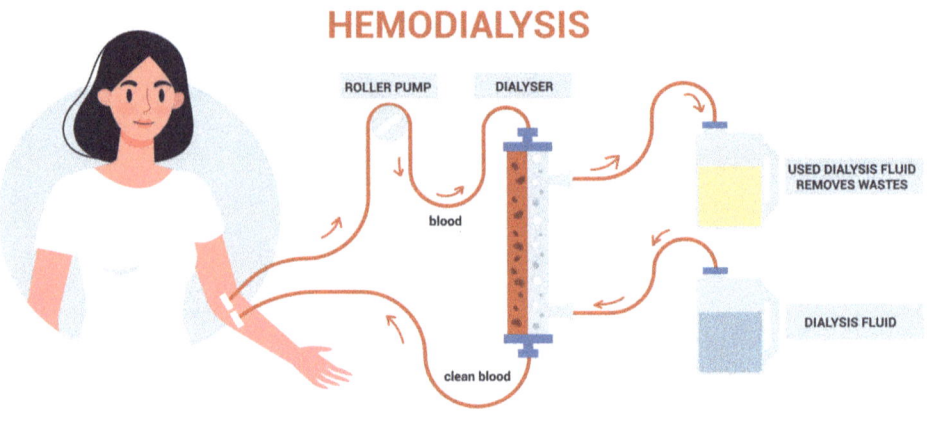

What is dialysis?	Dialysis is a treatment that takes over your kidney's function.
Two types of dialysis	*Hemodialysis*—uses a machine and a filter to remove waste products and water from the blood. Can be done at a dialysis facility or at home. *Peritoneal dialysis*—uses a fluid (dialysate) that is placed into the patient's abdominal cavity to remove waste products and fluid from the body.
Who needs dialysis?	A patient with kidney failure or chronic kidney disease. The two main causes of kidney failure and need for dialysis treatment are diabetes and high blood pressure. Dialysis needs to occur at least two to four times per week and appointments last several hours.

Renal failure	Renal failure occurs when there is a significant decrease or actual cessation of kidney function. Renal failure patients lose the ability to remove toxins from the blood, maintain fluid and electrolyte balance, control blood pressure, and produce red blood cells. As a result, these patients can develop congestive heart failure (due to fluid overload), electrolyte disorders, bleeding disorders, anemia, and symptoms related to toxin accumulation.

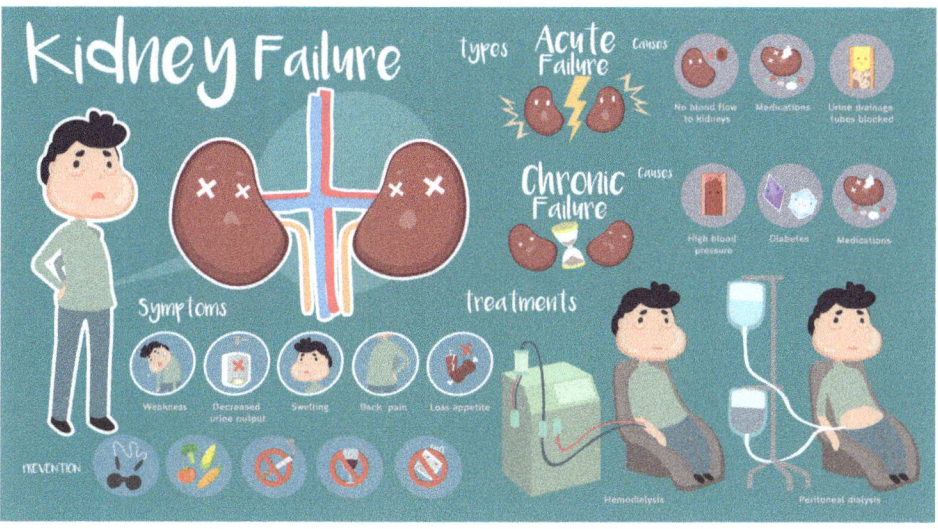

Signs and symptoms of renal failure	Early signs: - Lethargy - Swelling of the extremities - Abdominal pain - Decrease in urinary frequency Late signs: - Coma - Cardiac arrhythmias - Death

Renal Failure Complications

Uremia	Uremia is the term used to describe the signs and symptoms that are often present in a patient with inadequately treated renal failure. 　　Uremia can present with nausea, vomiting, diarrhea, weakness, dyspnea, irritated and itchy skin (pruritis), headache, and bruising or irregular darkening of the skin (hyperpigmentation). The treatment for uremia is dialysis.
Fluid overload	Fluid overload is caused by a reduction in the body's ability to excrete fluid through the urine. It may manifest as hypertension, peripheral edema, ascites, or pulmonary edema. The definitive treatment for fluid overload in a CRF patient is dialysis, but medications causing vascular dilation such as nitroglycerin can be used as a temporizing measure. Also, if the CRF patient has some residual renal function, diuretics can sometimes be helpful.

Anemia	Anemia is defined as a deficiency of hemoglobin (the oxygen-carrying material in red blood cells). Red blood cell production is stimulated by a protein produced in the kidneys called erythropoietin. As renal function decreases, erythropoietin secretion diminishes. Without erythropoietin, red blood cell production decreases, causing anemia. As a result, most patients with end-stage renal disease have anemia as a natural course of the disease.
Hypertension	The kidneys play a large part in blood pressure management. Almost all patients with kidney failure have hypertension. Many require multiple medications to control their blood pressure, but the definitive treatment for acute hypertension in these patients is dialysis.
Hyperkalemia	Hyperkalemia, or high potassium, is a common complication of renal failure. Malfunctioning kidneys are not able to effectively remove potassium from the body. With continued dietary intake of potassium, blood levels may increase. Patients may also present with hypokalemia (low potassium levels) if they are on an aggressive potassium, restricted diet, improperly dialyzed, or overuse loop diuretics without potassium supplementation.
Common ECG changes	The recognition and treatment of hyperkalemia are critical points for EMS providers to understand. Although renal failure patients can tolerate higher levels of potassium in their blood, hyperkalemia can lead to cardiac toxicity and cause fatal dysrhythmias if left untreated.

Peaked T waves widened QRS > .12 shortened QT interval ST segment depression	Calcium stabilizes the cardiac cell membranes but does not reduce potassium level in the blood while insulin, sodium bicarbonate, and beta agonists cause a reduction in serum potassium levels. Note that when insulin is used to reduce hyperkalemia, it must be given along with glucose to avoid causing hypoglycemia. We do not give insulin prehospital care; however, albuterol does reduce serum potassium levels and can be a safe and effective alternative for the treatment of hyperkalemia.
Coronary artery disease	Chronic diabetes rarely causes renal failure without also causing coronary artery disease and peripheral neuropathy (nerve degeneration). As a result, sensory nerves from the heart may not be fully functional and classic symptoms of myocardial ischemia, such as chest pain, may not be present. A high level of suspicion for acute coronary syndrome must be maintained in CRF patients.

Hyperkalemia ECG Strip

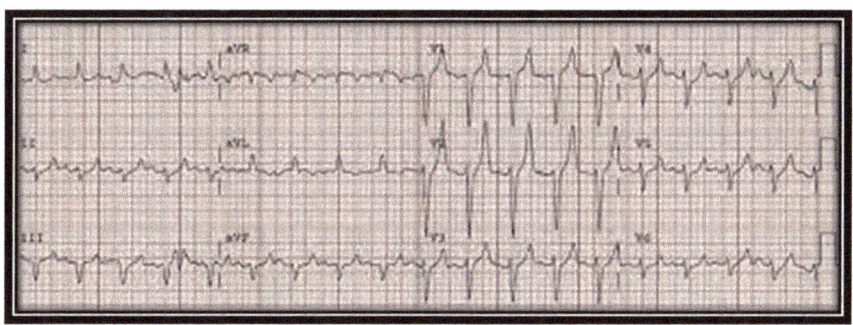

Electrolyte effects:

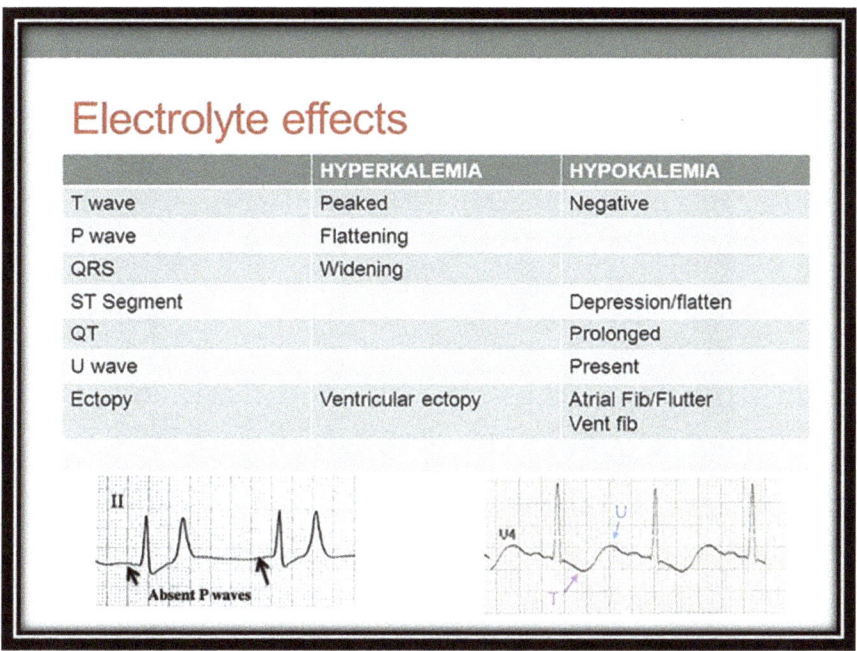

Chapter 31

ECG BASICS

Eight-Step Approach to ECG Interpretation

ECG
1. Rhythm Regular?
2. Heart Rate?
3. P waves?
4. PR Interval?
5. QRS Duration?
6. T wave?
7. Ectopic Beats?
8. Origin?
   } Identify Rhythm

1	*Determine the rate*—is it fast or slow? Tachycardia or bradycardia?
2	*Pattern of QRS complexes*—is it regular or irregular? Is it regularly irregular or irregularly irregular?
3	*QRS morphology*—narrow or wide complex? • *Narrow complex*—sinus, atrial, or junctional origin • *Wide complex*—ventricular origin or supraventricular with aberrant conduction
4	*P waves*—are they absent or present? • *Absent*—sinus arrest, atrial fibrillation • *Present*—morphology and PR interval may suggest sinus, atrial, junctional, or even retrograde from the ventricles *Measure the PR interval that should be 0.12–0.20 seconds (three to five small boxes).*
5	*Measure the QRS segment*—should be between 0.04–0.10 seconds. If you notice a prolonged QRS segment, it might be due to a bundle branch block that could be relatively benign or a sign of underlying heart disease.
6	*Observe the T wave.* The T wave represents repolarization (recovery) of the ventricles and should be upright in lead II and appear after the QRS segment. Any variations in the T waves are important to note. Inverted T waves could be due to a lack of oxygen to the heart, and too much potassium (hyperkalemia) could cause peaked T waves. Flat T waves may be due to too little potassium and a raised ST segment, and the end of the QRS segment to the beginning of the T wave might be due to a heart attack.

7	*Note any ectopic beats.* An ectopic beat is a change in a heart rhythm caused by beats arising from fibers outside the SA node, the normal impulse-generating system of the heart. If you notice ectopic beats, determine if they are premature atrial contractions (PACs), premature junctional contractions (PJCs), or premature ventricular contractions (PVCs). Also, note how many ectopic beats are present in the ECG, the interval at which they are appearing, their shape, and if they arise singularly or in groups.
8	*Determine the origin.* Determine where the rhythm is originating from. Key elements: - *Sinus.* 60–100 BPM, regular rhythm, P waves upright, round and present before each QRS segment, normal PR interval, and normal QRS duration. - *Atrial.* Rhythm may be regular or irregular and normal QRS segment but premature P waves and different shapes—flattened notched, peaked, inverted, or hidden. - *Junctional.* Look for a junctional type P wave—inverted before, during, or after the QRS segment that is normal in duration. - *Ventricular.* Wide and bizarre QRS segment and no P waves since the impulse is originating below the SA node. - *Paced rhythm.* Observe low voltage pacer spikes before the QRS.

Normal ECG Intervals

RR interval	0.6–1.2 second
P wave	80 milliseconds
PR interval	120–200 milliseconds
PR segment	50–120 milliseconds
QRS complex	80–100 milliseconds
J point	N/A
ST segment	80–120 milliseconds
T wave	160 milliseconds
ST interval	320 milliseconds
QT interval	420 milliseconds or less

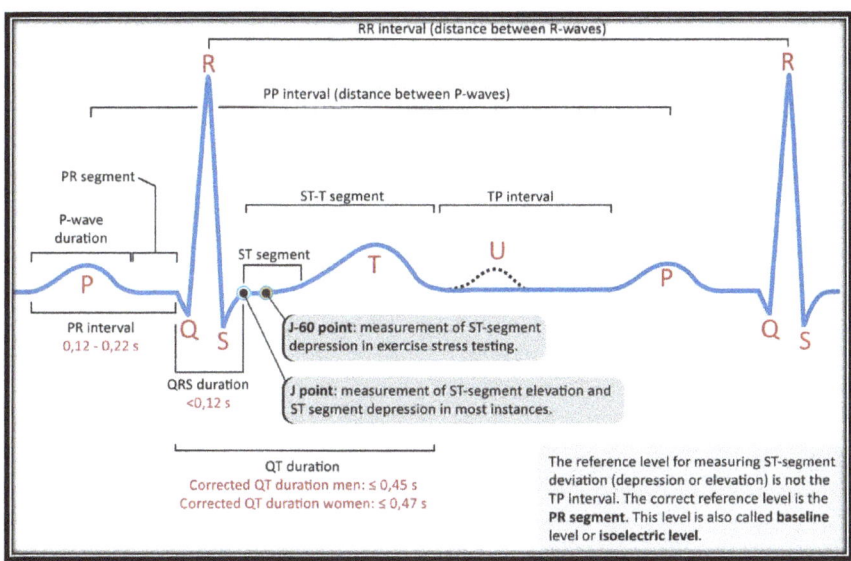

CHAPTER 32

HOME MEDS GUIDE

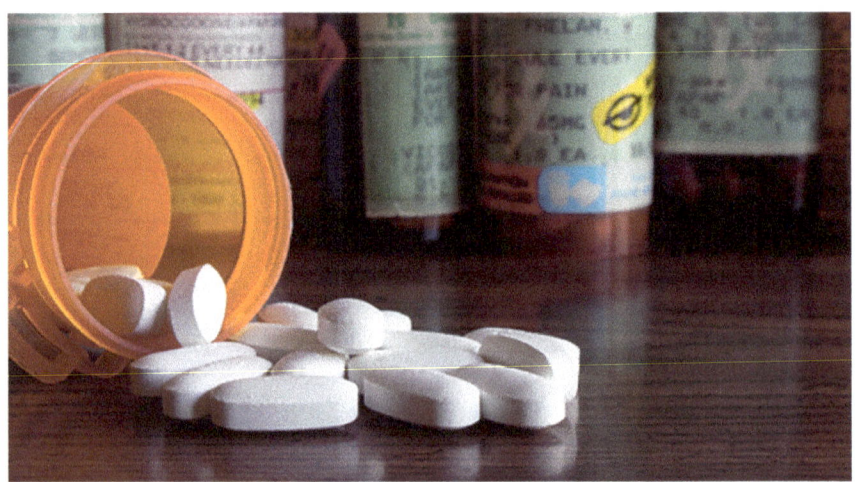

Drug Recognition Guide

As a student or medical provider, it can be difficult getting to know particular drugs and distinguishing between the various drug categories that you may be asked (under supervision) to administer.

This is a quick reference guide that can make it easier to recognize and remember drug names. Note: this is for general guidance only; it is not intended as a foolproof way to identify each and every drug in each and every drug category. Remember that there will always be exceptions to the rule. Nevertheless, the guide will be very useful while you are getting to know your drugs more thoroughly.

The drug names used in this guide refer to the drug's generic name as listed on the prescription sheet (and not to the drug's "brand name").

The color coding used in this guide is for ease of recognition purposes only and has no clinical significance. The guide lists more than 130 drugs subdivided into seventeen different categories.

One relatively easy way that can be used to help identify what group a particular drug belongs to is to look at the letters at the beginning (the prefix) or, more commonly, at the end (the suffix) of a generic drug's name. For example:

Ace inhibitors	Drugs used to treat hypertension, heart failure, diabetic nephropathy, or to reduce the likelihood of myocardial infarction. ACE (angiotensin-converting enzyme) inhibitors can be recognized by names that end with *pril.*	• Captopril • Cilazapril • Enalapril • Fosinopril • Lisinopril • Moexipril • Perindopril • Quinapril • Ramipril • Trandolapril

Alpha blockers	Drugs used to treat hypertension or urinary obstruction due to benign prostatic hyperplasia. Most (but not all) alpha blockers have names ending in *osin*.	• Alfuzosin • Doxazosin • Prazosin • Tamsulosin • Terazosin
Angiotensin II—receptor antagonists	Drugs used to treat hypertension, heart failure, or diabetic nephropathy end with sartan.	• Candesartan • Irbesartan • Losartan • Telmisartan • Valsartan
Antibiotics	Drugs used to treat bacterial infections with different kinds of antibiotic used to treat kinds of bacteria. Many antibiotics (including most antibiotics of the aminoglycoside, macrolide, and glycopeptide class) have names ending in *cin*. More specifically: antibiotics of the quinolone class end with *floxacin*,	• Amikacin • Amoxicillin • Ampicillin • Eefalexin • Eeftazidime • Ceftriaxone • Ciprofloxacin • Clarithromycin • Doripenem • Doxycycline • Erythromycin • Flucloxacillin • Gentamicin • Levofloxacin

penicillins can be identified by the suffix *cillin*, antibiotics of the cephalosporin class have names beginning with *cef*, carbapenem antibiotics end with *penem*, tetracycline antibiotics end with *cycline*, and rifamycin antibiotics have names beginning with *rif*.

- Lyme*cycline*
- Mero*penem*

Note a few exceptions: despite ending in *cin*, do not mistake ace*metacin* and indo*metacin* (NSAIDs), dari*fenacin* and soli*fenacin* (antimuscarinic drugs), or oxytocin (a drug used in

- Peni*cillin*
- Rifabutin
- Rifampi*cin*
- Tige*cycline*
- Vancomycin

Benzodiazipines	Sedatives given to treat insomnia, reduce anxiety, or to prevent or treat seizures. Most benzodiazepines have names ending with either *azepam* or *azolam*.	• Alprazolam • Clonazepam • Diazepam • Flurazepam • Loprazolam • Lorazepam • Lormetazepam • Midazolam • Nitrazepam • Oxazepam • Temazepam
Beta blockers	Drugs used to treat conditions such as hypertension, angina, heart failure, or cardiac arrhythmia and end with *lol* or *olol*.	• Atenolol • Bisoprolol

			• Esm*olol*
			• Meto*prolol*
			• Nebiv*olol*
			• Propran*olol*
			• Sota*lol*
	Bisphosphonates	Drugs used to treat osteoporosis or hypercalcemia—abnormally high levels of calcium in the blood. The drug inhibits bone reabsorption and so helps preserve bone density and prevent the release of excess calcium into the bloodstream. Bisphosphonates have names that end with *dronate* or *dronic acid*.	• Alen*dronic* acid • Clo*dronate* • Pami*dronate* • Rise*dronate* • Zole*dronic* acid

Class II—calcium channel blockers	Drugs used to treat hypertension or angina. Calcium channel blockers have names ending in *dipine*.	• Amlodipine • Felodipine • Isradipine • Lacidipine • Nicardipine • Nifedipine
Corticosteroids	Drugs given to reduce inflammation or to treat allergic, asthmatic, or rheumatic disorders. Most corticosteroids have names ending in *sone*, *solone*, *olone*, and *sonide*.	• Beclomethasone • Betamethasone • Budesonide • Circlesonide • Dexamethasone • Diflucortolone • Fludrocortisone • Flumetasone • Fluticasone • hydrocortisone • methylprednisolone

		• mometasone • prednisolone
5HT3 antagonists	Antiemetics used to treat severe nausea and vomiting and end with *setron*.	• Dolasetron • Granisetron • Ondansetron • Palonosetron
H2 blockers	Drugs used to treat esophageal reflux, dyspepsia, and gastric ulcers and end with the suffix *tidine*.	• Cimetidine • Famotidine • Nizatidine • Ranitidine
Nonsteroidal anti-inflammatory drugs (NSAIDs)	Anti-inflammatory painkillers that work by reducing prostaglandin levels. Many NSAIDs are derived from acetic acid, fenamic acid, or propionic acid and so tend to have names that end with *ac*, *fenac*, and *profen*.	• Aceclofenac • Dexibuprofen • Dexketoprofen • Diclofenac • Etodolac • Fenbufen • Fenoprofen • FFlurbiprofen • Ibuprofen • Ketoprofen • Ketorolac

Phenothiazines	Antipsychotic drugs developed in the 1950s to treat schizophrenia, but some of which are now also used as antiemetics—drugs to treat nausea and vomiting and end with either *promazine* or *perazine*.	• Chlor*promazine* • Levome*promazine* • Prochlor*perazine* • Trifluo*perazine*
Proton pump inhibitors (PPIs)	Drugs used to prevent or treat gastric or duodenal ulcers) have names ending in *prazole*.	• Esome*prazole* • Lanso*prazole* • Ome*prazole* • Panto*prazole* • Rabe*prazole*
Statins	Hypolipidaemic agents—drugs used to lower abnormally high levels of cholesterol in the blood. Statins end with the suffix *vastatin*.	• Ator*vastatin* • Flu*vastatin* • Pra*vastatin* • Rosu*vastatin* • Sim*vastatin*
Sulphonylureas	Drugs given to help treat type 2 diabetes. Most sulphonylureas can be recognized by names that begin with the prefix *gli*.	• Glibenclamide • Gliclazide • Glimepiride • Glipizide

Summary of Drug Prefixes and Suffixes

	Drug	Prefix/Suffix
1	Ace inhibitors	pril
2	Alpha blockers	osin
3	Antibiotics (many)	cin
4	Antibiotics (carbapenems)	penem
5	Antibiotics (cephalosporins)	cef
6	Antibiotics (penicillins)	cillin
7	Antibiotics (quinolones)	floxacin
8	Antibiotics (rifamycins)	rif
9	Antibiotics (tetracyclines)	cycline
10	Angiotensin-II receptor antagonists	sartan
11	Benzodiazepines	azepam or azolam
12	Beta blockers	lol or olol
13	Bisphosphonates	dronate or dronic acid
14	Class-II calcium channel blockers	dipine
15	Corticosteroids	sone, solone, olone, or sonide
16	5HT3 antagonists	setron
17	H2 blockers	tidine
18	NSAIDs (most)	ac, fenac, or profen
19	Phenothiazines	promazine or perazine

20	Proton pump inhibitors	prazole
21	Statins	vastatin
22	Sulphonylureas	gli

Chapter 33

EMS SKILL SHEETS

EMS Academy

BLS Skills Final Score Verification

Skill	Instructor Signature	Date	Score
Patient Assessment: Medical			
Patient Assessment: Trauma			
Vital Signs Assessment			
IV Setup and Med Assist (BLS)			
BLS Airway and Breathing Management			
Soft Tissue Injury: Bleeding Control			
12-Lead EKG Assessment			
Endotracheal Intubation and Ventilatory Management Assist			
Extra glottic Airway: King Tube			
Port-O2-Vent CPAP			

Flow-Safe II CPAP			
E-Z IO Intraosseous Infusion			
Adult BLS with AED			
Nebulizer Assembly			
Spinal Motion Restriction: Supine			
Spinal Motion Restriction: Seated/KED			
Traction Splint			
Obstetrical Emergencies: Childbirth			

Patient Assessment Medical

Name: Date: Start Time: End Time: Evaluator's Name:

Critical Failure Criteria in Bold	If Completed	Points Missed
1. Demonstrates body substance isolation precautions		AF
2. Determines scene is safe		AF

3.	Determines number and location of patients		
4.	Requests additional resources if necessary		
5.	Determines mechanism of injury/nature of illness		
6.	Verbalizes general impression of the patient (e.g. work of breathing, Skin signs, body position)		
7.	Determines chief complaint/ apparent life threats		
8.	Determines responsiveness (alert, responsive to verbal, responsive to pain, unresponsive)		AF
9. Airway: Assessment	Assessment Management (adjunct/suction)		AF
10. Breathing/ Ventilation	Assessment (rate/rhythm/ quality) Initiates appropriate oxygen therapy Assures adequate ventilation		AF
11. Circulation	Hemorrhage control Assess pulse (rate/rhythm/ quality) Assess		AF

	skin (color/ temperature/ moisture)		
12. Disability	Assess level of consciousness (person, place, time, event) Assess neuro function (circ./ sensory/motor x4)		AF
13. Investigates chief and associated complaint using appropriate assessment (e.g. OPQRST, PASTE, AEIOUTIPSS)			
Onset, Provokes, Quality, Radiates, Severity, Time	*Progression, associated chest pain, Sputum, Talk tolerance, Exercise tolerance*	*Alcohol, Epilepsy, Insulin, Overdose/ Oxygenation, Underdose/Uremia, Trauma, Infection, Psychosis, Stroke/Shock*	
14. Obtains baseline vital signs (to include BP, HR, RR, lung sounds, pupils, ECG, pulse ox, and/or blood glucose if appropriate)			
15. Correctly performs Cincinnati Pre-Hospital Stroke Scale if indicated			AF
16. Obtains past medical history			
17. Obtains list of allergies			
18. Obtains list of current medications			

19. Continuous reassessment, including vital signs		AF
Total Points		100

Critical Fail Criteria

- Failure to manage the patient as a competent EMT.
- Exhibits unacceptable affect with patient or other personnel.
- Uses or orders a dangerous or inappropriate intervention.
- Failure to obtain baseline BP, HR, and RR.
- Failure to complete skill assessment within ten minutes.

Evaluator's Signature: Date:

Patient Assessment
Trauma

Name: Date: Start Time: End Time: Evaluator's Name:

Critical Failure Criteria in Bold	If Completed	Points Missed
1. Demonstrates body substance isolation precautions		AF
2. Determines scene is safe		AF
3. Determines the number and location of patients		
4. Requests additional resources if necessary		
5. Determines mechanism of injury/nature of illness		

6. Considers/takes spinal motion restriction			AF
7. Verbalizes general impression of the patient			
8. Determines chief complaint/ apparent life threats			
9. Determines responsiveness (alert, responsive to verbal, responsive to pain, unresponsive)			AF
10. Airway: Assessment	Assessment Management (adjunct/suction)		AF
11. Breathing/ Ventilation	Assessment (rate/rhythm/quality) Initiates appropriate oxygen therapy Assures adequate ventilation Manages injuries (exposes/palpates thorax)		AF
12. Circulation	Hemorrhage control Assess pulse (rate/rhythm/quality) Assess skin (color/temperature/moisture)		AF

13. Disability	Assess level of consciousness (person, place, time, event) Assess neuro function (circ./sensory/motor x4)		AF
14. Expose	Exposes patient Prevent heat loss with blanket		AF
15. Patient packaging: Complete spinal motion restriction if indicated			
16. Initiate's transport for critical patients within 10-minute time limit			AF
17. Attempts to obtain SAMPLE history			
18. Assess the head	Inspects and palpates the scalp and ears Assess eyes (pupils equal, round, reactive to light) Assess the face, including oral and nasal areas		

19. Assess the neck	Inspects and palpates the cervical spine Assess for jugular vein distension Assess for tracheal deviation		
20. Assess the chest	Inspects, palpates Auscultates as needed		
21. Assess the abdomen/ pelvis	Assess the abdomen Assess the pelvis Verbalizes assessment of genitalia/ perineum		
22. Assess extremities	Inspects and palpates all four extremities. assessing motor, sensory and circulatory function		
23. Assess posterior	Assesses posterior thorax Assesses lumbar and buttocks		
24. Obtains baseline vital signs (to include BP, HR, and RR)			
25. Manages secondary injuries appropriately			

	If Completed	Points Missed
26. Verbalizes reassessment, including vital signs		
Total Points		100

Critical Fail Criteria

- Failure to manage the patient as a competent EMT.
- Exhibits unacceptable affect with patient or other personnel.
- Uses or orders a dangerous or inappropriate intervention.
- Failure to complete skill assessment within ten minutes.

Evaluator's Signature: Date:

Vital Signs Assessment

Name: Date: Start Time: End Time: Evaluator's Name:

Critical Failure Criteria in Bold	If Completed	Points Missed
1. Demonstrates body substance isolation precautions		AF
Pulse		
2. Selects pulse site Adult: Radial, brachial, carotid, femoral Pediatric: Brachial, carotid, femoral, apical		
3. Locates and palpates pulse		
4. Determines accurate pulse rate		AF
5. Determines quality of pulse: regular/irregular, strong/weak		

Respirations		
6. Observes/palpates rise and fall of chest or abdomen		
7. Determines accurate respiration rate		AF
8. Determines effort and regularity of respirations		
Blood Pressure: Palpated		
9. Applies cuff appropriately to patient: on bare skin, artery line placed appropriately, cuff sized appropriately		
10. Palpates radial or brachial artery		
11. Inflates cuff to at least 20mm Hg above the point where pulse is lost		
12. Slowly deflates cuff		
13. Determines accurate systolic blood pressure when pulse returns		AF
Blood Pressure: Auscultated		
14. Applies cuff appropriately to patient: on bare skin, artery marker placed appropriately, cuff sized appropriately		
15. Locates brachial artery		
16. With stethoscope earpieces placed appropriately, places diaphragm over brachial artery site		

17. Inflates cuff to at least 20mmHg above palpated pressure		
18. Slowly deflates cuff		
19. Determines accurate systolic and diastolic blood pressure		AF
Total Points		100

Critical Fail Criteria

- Failure to manage the patient as a competent EMT.
- Exhibits unacceptable affect with patient or other personnel.
- Uses or orders a dangerous or inappropriate intervention.
- Not within +/- 4 beats of monitor during pulse assessment.
- Not within +/- 6 mmHg of monitor during blood pressure assessment.
- Not within +/- 2 respirations of monitor during respiration assessment.
- Failure to complete skill assessment within ten minutes.

Evaluator's Signature: Date:

IV Setup and Med Assist (BLS)

Name: Date: Start Time: End Time: Evaluator's Name:

Critical Failure Criteria in Bold	If Completed	Points Missed
1. Demonstrates body substance isolation precautions		AF
2. Confirms that the solution is appropriate, clear, not expired		

3. Selects appropriate IV tubing (i.e. 60 drop set vs. 10 drop set)		
4. Closes roller clamp		
5. Removes protective caps from the IV bag and tubing without contamination		
6. Inserts IV tubing into correct port using aseptic technique; maintains aseptic technique throughout procedure		AF
7. Squeezes drip chamber until half-full of solution		
8. Opens roller clamp		
9. Allows fluid to run through tubing, expelling all the air		
10. Closes roller clamp. Advises Paramedic that IV solution is ready		
Medication Administration		
11. Correctly identifies and selects requested medication within 10 seconds		
Total Points		100

Critical Fail Criteria

- Failure to manage the patient as a competent EMT.
- Exhibits unacceptable affect with patient or other personnel.
- Uses or orders a dangerous or inappropriate intervention.

- Failure to attach IV tubing to IV bag and flood tubing with aseptic technique.
- Failure to ensure aseptic technique.
- Failure to correctly identify appropriate med and administration set.
- Failure to complete skill assessment within ten minutes.
- Failure to properly spike bag.
- Failure to expel air from IV line.

Evaluator's Signature: Date:

BLS Airway and Breathing Management

Name: Date: Start Time: End Time: Evaluator's Name:

Critical Failure Criteria in Bold	If completed	Points Missed
1. Demonstrates body substance isolation precautions		AF
Oxygen Administration		

2. Attaches regulator to oxygen tank.
   a. Ensures O-ring is in place
   b. Tightens regulator to tank securely with hand only
   c. Determines that regulator is in "off" position		

3. Opens main valve at least 1 turn
   a. Checks pressure on regulator
   b. Checks for leaks		

4. Attaches nasal cannula properly; target oxygen saturation is 94-95%
    a. Places prongs correctly in nose, tightens tubing around ears
    b. Sets liter flow between 2 and 6 liters per minute		

5. Attaches non-rebreather properly, target oxygen saturation is 94-95%
    a. Non-Rebreather: fills reservoir, properly fits mask around nose and mouth
    b. Sets liter flow between 10 and 15 liters per minute		

6. Reassess patient's respiratory status for improvement		
7. Turns off regulator		
Nasopharyngeal Airway		
1. Determines correct size of nasopharyngeal airway (measures from tip of earlobe to tip of nose)		
2. Lubricates nasopharyngeal airway with water-based lubricant		
3. Inserts nasopharyngeal airway into either nare with bevel toward septum, pushing posteriorly, rotating as appropriate so that NPA curves inferiorly		

Oropharyngeal Airway			
1.	Determines correct size of oropharyngeal airway (measures from Angle of the jaw to corner of mouth)		
2.	Inserts oropharyngeal airway toward roof of the mouth until resistance is met, then rotates airway 180 degrees. Continues until flange meets lips.		
Bag Valve Mask			
1.	Attaches bag valve mask to oxygen tank		
2.	Sets regulator flow to 15 liters per minute		
3.	Opens airway with head tilt, chin lift or modified jaw thrust, if indicated		
4.	Creates tight seal between mask and face using CE clamp technique		

5.	Ventilates patient steadily
	   a. Observes for chest rise and fall
	   b. Checks for gastric distention
	   c. Checks for leaks around face and mask, repositions as necessary		

6.	Ventilates patient at appropriate rate (adult: 1 breath every 6 seconds; infant: 1 breath every 3-5 seconds)		

7.	Reassesses ventilatory status		
Flexible (Soft) Suction Catheter			
1.	Prepares suction equipment: connects catheter and tubing to suction unit		
2.	Test's suction for vacuum, sets strength for adult (100) or child (80)		

3.	Determines depth of catheter insertion
	   a. Nose - tip of nose to tip of earlobe
	   b. Mouth - tip of earlobe to corner of mouth		

4.	Insert's catheter into patient to measured depth		
5.	Initiate's vacuum, suctions while withdrawing catheter, maximum 15 seconds		
6.	Reassesses ventilatory status		
Rigid (Hard) Suction Catheter (Yankauer)			
1.	Determines depth of catheter insertion (measures from tip of earlobe to corner of mouth)		
2.	Insert's catheter into patient's mouth to measured depth		
3.	Initiate's vacuum, suctions while withdrawing catheter, maximum 15 seconds		
4.	Reassesses ventilatory status		
Total Points			100

Critical Fail Criteria

- Failure to manage the patient as a competent EMT.
- Exhibits unacceptable affect with patient or other personnel.
- Uses or orders a dangerous or inappropriate intervention.
- Failure to complete skill assessment within ten minutes.
- Failure to physically perform skill assessment.

Evaluator's Signature: Date:

Soft Tissue Injury: Bleeding Control

Name: Date: Start Time: End Time: Evaluator's Name:

Critical Failure Criteria in Bold	If completed	Points Missed
1. Demonstrates body substance isolation precautions		AF
2. Applies direct pressure to the wound		
The examiner now informs the candidate that the wound continues to bleed		
3. Applies tourniquet with proper technique (including placement of tourniquet closest to joint <u>most</u> proximal to patient's core)		AF
4. Tightens tourniquet until bleeding is stopped or controlled		
5. Documents on tourniquet or patient, date and time tourniquet applied		

The examiner now informs the candidate that bleeding is controlled		
6. Assures wound now bandaged appropriately		
The examiner must now inform the candidate the patient is now showing signs and symptoms indicative of hypoperfusion		
7. Applies oxygen as indicted		AF
8. Initiates steps to prevent heat loss from the patient		AF
9. Indicates the need for immediate transport		AF
Total Points		100

Critical Fail Criteria

- Failure to manage the patient as a competent EMT.
- Exhibits unacceptable affect with patient or other personnel.
- Uses or orders a dangerous or inappropriate intervention.
- Failure to apply tourniquet with proper technique and placement.
- Failure to tighten tourniquet until bleeding stops or is controlled.
- Failure to treat signs of hypoperfusion.
- Failure to verbalize need for immediate transport.
- Failure to complete skill assessment within ten minutes.

Evaluator's Signature: Date:

12-Lead EKG Assessment

Name: Date: Start Time: End Time: Evaluator's Name:

Critical Failure Criteria in Bold	If Completed	Points Missed
1. Demonstrates body substance isolation precautions		AF
Examiner asks for 8 indications for 12-lead EKG		

2. Verbalizes indications (must get at least 8):
  a. sub-sternal chest pain
  b. discomfort or tightness radiating to jaw, left shoulder or arm
  c. nausea
  d. diaphoresis
  e. dyspnea
  f. anxiety
  g. syncope/dizziness
  h. "suspicious" symptoms
  i. paramedic judgement
  j. treating patient for any protocol which specifies need for 12-lead ECG (e.g. ROSC, dysrhythmias, CVA, etc.)
  k. significant history of cardiac or known risk factors (e.g. hypertension, diabetes, etc.)		

3.	Places all four limb leads in symmetric fashion in correct location.		AF
4.	Prepares patient for chest lead placement a. Verbalizes need to shave and/or clean skin, begins monitoring patient		
5.	Place and verbalizes 12 lead electrodes in correct locations: a. V-1: right 4th intercostal space at sternal border b. V-2: left 4th intercostal space at sternal border c. V-3: halfway between V2 and V4 d. V-4: left 5th intercostal space, mid-clavicular line e. V-5: horizontal to V4, anterior axillary line f. V-6: horizontal to V5, mid-axillary line g. V-4R: right 5th intercostal space, mid-clavicular line (use in all suspected inferior MI's for establishing appropriateness for administering nitroglycerin or morphine)		AF
6.	Locates "12-lead" indicator on screen and presses button. a. Student correctly enters patient age and gender, and acquires 12-lead		

7. If the paramedic identifies a STEMI, the patient must be transported to the nearest STAR receiving hospital, or the STAR facility of the patient's choice.		
8. Indicates need for early receiving hospital notification with clear warning that a. "STEMI Alert" patient is en route.		
9. Indicates need to acquire repeat 12 lead tracings during transport. All tracings should be saved.		
Total Points		**100**

Critical Fail Criteria

- Failure to manage the patient as a competent EMT.
- Exhibits unacceptable affect with patient or other personnel.
- Uses or orders a dangerous or inappropriate intervention.
- Failure to properly place limb leads and/or failure to properly place IV-leads.
- Failure to complete skill assessment within ten minutes.

Evaluator's Signature: Date:

Endotracheal Intubation and Ventilatory Management Assist

Name: Date: Start Time: End Time: Evaluator's Name:

Critical Failure Criteria in Bold	If Completed	Points Missed
1. Demonstrates body substance isolation precautions		AF
2. Opens the airway manually using head tilt/chin lift, or jaw thrust if trauma is suspected		
3. Elevates tongue, properly inserts BLS adjunct (oropharyngeal or nasopharyngeal airway)		
Examiner now informs candidate that no gag reflex is present, and patient accepts adjunct		
4. Attaches oxygen reservoir to bag valve mask and connects to high flow oxygen (12-15 liters per minute)		AF
5. Ventilates patient at a rate of 10 per minute, with appropriate volumes		AF
Examiner now informs candidate that pulse oximetry is 85%; and patient will be intubated		
6. Identifies/selects proper equipment for intubation. Checks for: a. Proper tube size b. Cuff leaks		

c. Laryngoscope bulb operational (white, bright, tight)		
7. Removes oropharyngeal airway and positions head properly		
Examiner intubates patient/mannequin		
8. Properly ventilates patient		
9. Confirms placement by bilateral lung auscultation and over epigastrium		AF
10. Verbalize at least one additional method to confirm proper tube placement		
11. Zeroes capnography on monitor		AF
12. Attaches capnography to endotracheal tube appropriately		AF
13. Verbalizes normal capnography range (35-45 mmHg) and how to correct abnormal readings		
14. Secures endotracheal tube (may be verbalized)		
Total Points		100

Critical Fail Criteria

- Failure to manage the patient as a competent EMT.
- Exhibits unacceptable affect with patient or other personnel.
- Uses or orders a dangerous or inappropriate intervention.

- Failure to start ventilations within 30 seconds of body substance isolation, or interrupts ventilations for more than thirty seconds at any time.
- Failure to take or verbalize body substance isolation precautions.
- Failure to voice and ultimately provide high oxygen concentration.
- Failure to ventilate patient at a rate of ten/minute.
- Failure to attach capnography.
- Failure to complete skill assessment within ten minutes.

Evaluator's Signature: Date:

Extraglottic Airway

KingTube

Name: Date: Start Time: End Time: Evaluator's Name:

Critical Failure Criteria in Bold	If Completed	Points Missed
1. Demonstrates body substance isolation precautions		AF
2. Opens the airway manually using head tilt/ chin lift unless trauma		
3. Properly measures and inserts simple adjunct (oropharyngeal o r nasopharyngeal airway)		
Examiner now informs candidate no gag reflex is present and patient accepts adjunct		

4.	Attaches oxygen reservoir to bag valve mask and connects to high flow oxygen (12-15 L/min)		AF
5.	Ventilates patient at a rate of 10 breaths/minute (adult) or 12-20 breaths/minute (pediatric) with appropriate volumes		AF
Examiner states pulse oximetry is 85%, and King Tube is to be inserted. Examiner asks candidate, "What are the indications and contraindications for using a King Tube?"			
6.	Verbalizes INDICATIONS: a. BLS airway not adequate b. Unconscious and without purposeful movement c. No gag reflex d. Apnea		
7.	Verbalizes CONTRAINDICATIONS: a. Gag reflex, b. History of esophageal disease or varices, c. Ingestion of caustics		
8.	Identifies/selects proper size King LTD based on height		AF
Examiner inserts King Tube into patient/mannequin			
9.	Confirms placement by bilateral lung auscultation and over epigastrium		AF
10.	Verbalizes at least one additional method to confirm proper placement		

11. Installs capnography adapter and attaches to King tube		AF
12. Readjusts cuff inflation to seal volume of esophagus as needed		
13. Secures King Tube with commercial device		
Total Points		100

Critical Fail Criteria

- Failure to manage the patient as a competent EMT.
- Exhibits unacceptable affect with patient or other personnel.
- Uses or orders a dangerous or inappropriate intervention.
- Failure to complete skill assessment within ten minutes.

Evaluator's Signature: Date:

Tube Color	Tube Size	Height	LBRT
Green	#2	35" to 45"	Yellow
Orange	#2.5	41" to 51"	Blue
Yellow	#3	4' to 5'	Green
Red	#4	5' to 6'	N/A
Purple	#5	> 6'	N/A

Nasotracheal Intubation

Name: Date: Start Time: End Time: Evaluator's Name:

Critical Failure Criteria in Bold	If Completed	Points Missed
1. Demonstrates body substance isolation precautions		AF
2. Ventilates patient with 100% oxygen using bag valve mask		AF
3. Explains procedure to patient		
4. Pretreats both nares with Phenylephrine HCL .25% nasal spray		
5. Administers Cetacaine spray to the posterior pharynx		
6. Lubricates NPA with 2% Lidocaine gel and inserts into larger nare		
7. Chooses correct size ET tube, removes stylet, attaches BAAM whistle, lubricates tube with 2% Lidocaine gel		
8. Place's patient in sniffing position		
9. Removes NPA		
10. Inserts ETT into pre-selected nare, uses gentle twisting motion until it passes the turbinates' and listens for BAAM whistle as tube approaches glottic opening		

11. Advances distal end of tube rapidly into the glottic opening as patient inhales. BAAM whistle should be loud and clear.		AF
12. Inflates distal cuff with 10-12 ml of air, until balloon is firm		
13. Removes BAAM whistle		
14. Ventilates the patient with 100% oxygen via BVM		AF
15. Confirms tube placement by (must get capnography and at least two others): a. Capnography* b. Observing equal chest rise and fall c. Auscultating lung fields and epigastric area d. Misting or fogging in tube		AF
16. Secures tube with tape.		
17. Reconfirms tube placement every 5 minutes or any movement of the patient.		AF
18. Completes procedure in 90 seconds or less		
Total Points		100

Critical Fail Criteria

- Failure to manage the patient as a competent EMT.
- Exhibits unacceptable affect with patient or other personnel.
- Uses or orders a dangerous or inappropriate intervention.
- Unrecognized esophageal placement.

- Failure to confirm tube placement.
- Failure to reconfirm tube placement.
- Failure to complete skill assessment within ten minutes.

Evaluator's Signature: Date:

Port-O$_2$-Vent CPAP

Name: Date: Start Time: End Time: Evaluator's Name:

Critical Failure Criteria in Bold	If Completed	Points Missed
1. Demonstrates body substance isolation precautions		AF
2. Oxygen therapy initiated via assisted bag valve mask or high flow O$_2$		AF
Examiner asks for four indications for use of CPAP		
3. Verbalizes indications (must verbalize at least 4): a. Age 8 or older, and in moderate to severe respiratory distress b. Congestive heart failure with pulmonary edema c. Acute exacerbation of chronic obstructive pulmonary disease or asthma d. Near drowning e. GCS 14 or above f. O$_2$ saturation < 94%		AF

Examiner asks for three contraindications for use of CPAP			

4. Verbalizes contraindications (must verbalize at least 3):
   a. Maxillo-facial or chest trauma with potential for pneumothorax
   b. Epistaxis, active vomiting, or gastrointestinal bleeding
   c. Apnea, cardiac arrest
   d. Tracheostomy
   e. Systolic blood pressure of less than 90 mmHg
		AF	

5. Secures adequate oxygen source for CPAP (minimum 1,000 psi available)
   a. Uses a "D" cylinder, or
   b. Uses quick-connect fitting at wall oxygen outlet in ambulance			

6. Attaches green oxygen supply line to oxygen source (regulator or wall outlet) and to the CPAP unit			
7. Attaches clear plastic CPAP supply line to unit. Rotates connector right t o lock in place			

8. Attaches appropriate size mask to CPAP supply line. Verbalize 3 sizes
   a. Small
   b. Regular (used in most patients)
   c. Large			

9. Attaches HEPA filter to face mask assembly		
10. Set's delivery pressure on CPAP unit to zero		
11. Turns on O_2 supply tank at regulator; assures regulator's liter flow is set to "off"		
12. Rotates dial on CPAP unit ½ turn to supply low pressure O_2 delivery to mask		
13. Explains CPAP to the patient, and how it will help the patient to breathe		
14. Applies mask to patient's face and encourages patient to breathe normally		
15. Adjusts pressure to proper setting between 7.5-10.0 cm H2O		AF
16. As patient learns to breathe with mask held in place, attaches the head strap using the four posts on the mask		
17. Reassess patient for signs of improvement or deterioration		
18. Confirms nasal mask fit and checks for leaks during any movement or manipulation; adjusts as necessary		

19. Prepares for transport and verbalizes need to make early hospital notification of transport of patients on CPAP: *"This is a CPAP patient."*		
Examiner states that patient is becoming fatigued.		
20. If patient becomes too fatigued to trigger CPAP, or becomes unconscious, discontinues CPAP and continues with assisted ventilation using a BVM and/or intubates		AF
21. At hospital, does not discontinue CPAP until appropriately replaced by respiratory therapy, such as CPAP or BiPAP		
Total Points		100

Critical Fail Criteria

- Failure to manage the patient as a competent EMT.
- Exhibits unacceptable affect with patient or other personnel.
- Uses or orders a dangerous or inappropriate intervention.
- Failure to properly assemble CPAP unit.
- Failure to complete skill assessment within ten minutes.

Evaluator's Signature: Date:

Flow-Safe II CPAP

Name: Date: Start Time: End Time: Evaluator's Name:

Critical Failure Criteria in Bold	If Completed	Points Missed
1. Demonstrates body substance isolation precautions		**AF**
2. Oxygen therapy initiated via assisted bag valve mask or high flow O_2		**AF**
Examiner asks for four indications for use of CPAP		

3. Verbalizes indications (must verbalize at least 4):
  a. Age 8 or older, and in moderate to severe respiratory distress
  b. Congestive heart failure with pulmonary edema
  c. Acute exacerbation of chronic obstructive pulmonary disease or asthma
  d. Near drowning
  e. GCS 14 or above
  f. O_2 saturation < 94%
		AF

Examiner asks for three contraindications for use of CPAP		
4. Verbalizes contraindications (must verbalize at least 3): a. Maxillo-facial or chest trauma with potential for pneumothorax		**AF**

	b. Epistaxis, active vomiting, or gastrointestinal bleeding c. Apnea, cardiac arrest d. Tracheostomy e. Systolic blood pressure of less than 90 mmHg		
5.	Secures adequate oxygen source for CPAP (minimum 1,000 psi available) a. Uses a "D" cylinder, or b. Uses wall oxygen outlet in ambulance		
6.	Attach Flow-Safe II to regulator or flowmeter		
7.	Loosen Velcro straps, and pulls head harness back over the mask		
8.	Turn oxygen flow rate to 10 liters per minute		
9.	Explains CPAP to the patient, and how it will help the patient to breathe		
10.	Applies mask to patient's face and encourages patient to breathe normally		
11.	Adjusts pressure to proper setting between 7.5 to 10.0 cm H2O		**AF**
12.	As patient learns to breathe with mask held in place, attaches the h e a d harness and adjusts Velcro straps (mask should be airtight)		

13. Administer a nebulizer treatment by turning control knob to green		
14. Titrates liters/minute flow to maintain pressure, using manometer as a guide		
15. Measure capnography during CPAP application		
16. Reassess patient for signs of improvement or deterioration		
17. Confirms nasal mask fit and checks for leaks during any movement or manipulation; adjusts as necessary		
18. Prepares for transport and verbalizes need to make early hospital notification of transport of patients on CPAP: *"This is a CPAP patient."*		
Examiner states that patient is becoming fatigued		
19. If patient becomes too fatigued to trigger CPAP, or becomes unconscious, discontinues CPAP and continues with assisted ventilation using a BVM and/or intubates		**AF**
20. At hospital, does not discontinue CPAP until appropriate replacement by Respiratory therapy, such as CPAP or BiPAP		
Total Points		100

Critical Fail Criteria

- Failure to manage the patient as a competent EMT.
- Exhibits unacceptable affect with patient or other personnel.
- Uses or orders a dangerous or inappropriate intervention.
- Failure to properly assemble CPAP unit.
- Failure to complete skill assessment within ten minutes.

Evaluator's Signature: Date:

Flow (liters/minute)	CPAP Pressure: Neb OFF	CPAP Pressure: Neb ON
6	2.0–3.0	1.0–2.0
10	6.0–7.0	2.0–3.0
12	8.0–9.0	3.0–4.0
15	11.0–12-.0	4.0–5.0

CPAP Pressure	Liters/minute: Neb OFF	Liters/minute: Neb ON
5.0	8–9	15–16
7.5	10–12	19–20
10.0	13–14	24–25
13.0 (max)	flush	28–30

Needle Thoracostomy/Needle Decompression

Name: Date: Start Time: End Time: Evaluator's Name:

Critical Failure Criteria in Bold	If Completed	Points Missed
1. Demonstrates body substance isolation precautions		AF
2. Oxygenates patient as indicated and appropriately		AF

3. Verbalizes indications (must get at least 5):
   a. Decreased breath sounds, unilaterally or bilaterally
   b. Tracheal shift away from affected side
   c. Extreme dyspnea
   d. Hypotension (weak or/absent radial pulse)
   e. Tachycardia
   f. Agitation
   g. Jugular vein distension
		AF

4. Removes providine swab, provided pleural decompression needle (10g, 3"), 30cc syringe, dressing and tape from the pleural decompression kit		

5. Locates appropriate site:
   a. 2nd intercostal space, mid-clavicular line (primary)
   b. 4th or 5th intercostal space, mid-axillary line (secondary)
		AF

6. Prepares patient by swabbing the identified site with providine or alcohol prep		
7. Attaches needle to 30cc syringe, always keeping the needle sterile.		AF
8. Inserts the needle over the superior aspect of 3rd rib into the 2nd intercostal space (mid-clavicular), or over the superior aspect of 5th or 6th rib into the 4th or 5th intercostal space (mid-axillary).		AF
9. Slowly advance needle until entrance into pleural space (verified by a "pop" or lack of resistance).		
10. Advance the needle and catheter slightly further to ensure catheter has entered the pleural space. Hold needle and advance catheter until hub rests against skin. Withdraw needle and dispose into sharps container.		AF
11. Secures one-way valve or stopcock to the catheter and secures catheter hub to the patient with tape		
12. Reassesses patient for improvement in respiratory status, including radial pulse, blood pressure, respiration rate		
Total Points		100

Critical Fail Criteria

- Failure to manage the patient as a competent EMT.
- Exhibits unacceptable affect with patient or other personnel.
- Uses or orders a dangerous or inappropriate intervention.
- Failure to complete skill assessment within ten minutes.

Evaluator's Signature: Date:

EZ-IO Intraosseous Infusion

Name: Date: Start Time: End Time: Evaluator's Name:

Critical Failure Criteria in Bold	If Completed	Points Missed
1. Demonstrates body substance isolation precautions		AF
Examiner asks for four indications for use of EZ-IO		
2. Verbalizes indications (must get at least 4): a. Unable to obtain a pulse b. Unresponsive c. Apneic d. Hypotension with shock e. Acute deteriorating level of consciousness f. Unable to obtain peripheral IV access after 2 attempts (critical patients only)		AF
Examiner asks for three contraindications for use of EZ-IO		

3. Verbalizes contraindications (must get at least 3):
   a. Fractured to bone and/or splint distal to insertion site
   b. Prior orthopedic procedures such as knee replacement, amputation
   c. Previous IO attempt in same extremity
   d. Preexisting condition affecting extremity such as burn/infection
   e. Routine IV access obtainable (non-critical patients)
		AF

4. Selects appropriate equipment to include:
   a. EZ IO Driver
   b. Small (pink) Medium (blue) and Large (Yellow) IO needle
   c. EZ IO extension set
   d. 2% Lidocaine
   e. <10ml normal saline flush (conscious), 5ml normal saline flush (unconscious)
   f. Alcohol or other approved iodine based disinfectant swab
   g. IV bag normal saline, tubing		

5. Identifies proper anatomical site for IO puncture:
   a. Proximal medial tibia – 2-3 cm below tuberosity (primary site), or
   b. Humeral head (secondary, if tibia site is unavailable)
		AF

Examiner inserts IO at selected site		
6. Secures IO with approved devices and reassesses patient a. If humeral head insertion is chosen, applies sling and swath		
7. Attaches IV line and pressure infuser		
8. If infiltration occurs: stop infusion, remove needle, apply pressure bandage		
Total Points		100

Critical Fail Criteria

- Failure to manage the patient as a competent EMT
- Exhibits unacceptable affect with patient or other personnel
- Uses or orders a dangerous or inappropriate intervention
- Failure to complete skill assessment within ten minutes

Evaluator's Signature: Date:

Adult BLS with AED

Name: Date: Start Time: End Time: Evaluator's Name:

Critical Failure Criteria in Bold	If Completed	Points Missed
1. Demonstrates body substance isolation precautions		AF
2. Assesses patient response and breathing status (at least 5 seconds, no more than 10 seconds)		
3. Checks for carotid pulse (at least 5 seconds, no more than 10 seconds)		

4. Gives five cycles of high-quality CPR
  a. Given at a ratio of 30 compressions to 2 breaths
  b. Hands placed correctly (heel of one hand on lower third of sternum, other hand stacked and interlaced on the first)
  c. Compresses at rate between 100 and 120 per minute (gives c o mpressions in 15 to 18 seconds)
  d. Compresses at depth between 2" and 2.4" (at least 23 out of 30)
  e. Allows full chest recoil (at least 23 out of 30)
		AF

f. Gives 2 breaths with bag valve mask in less than 10 seconds		
Examiner tells student that AED has arrived		
5. Applies pads to patient appropriately		
6. Turns on AED and presses analyze		
7. If AED indicates shock, clears patient, and delivers shock		
8. Immediately resumes high quality CPR		
Total Points		100

Critical Fail Criteria

- Failure to manage the patient as a competent EMT.
- Exhibits unacceptable affect with patient or other personnel.
- Uses or orders a dangerous or inappropriate intervention.
- Failure to complete skill assessment within ten minutes.
- Interruption of CPR greater than ten seconds (not including AED analyze).

Evaluator's Signature: Date:

Nebulizer Assembly: ALS Assist

Name: Date: Start Time: End Time: Evaluator's Name:

Critical Failure Criteria in Bold	If completed	Points Missed
1. Demonstrates body substance isolation precautions		AF
2. Knows location, contents, and layout of albuterol nebulizer set-up		
3. Assembles nebulizer in hand-held configuration (including oxygen)		
4. Assembles nebulizer in mask configuration (including oxygen)		
5. Assembles nebulizer in bag valve mask configuration (including oxygen)		
6. Keeps nebulizer chamber positioned properly while bagging patient		
7. Assembles nebulizer in CPAP configuration (including oxygen)		
8. Keeps nebulizer chamber positioned properly while CPAP engaged		
9. Reassesses patient.		
Total Points		100

Critical Fail Criteria

- Failure to manage the patient as a competent EMT.
- Exhibits unacceptable affect with patient or other personnel.
- Uses or orders a dangerous or inappropriate intervention.
- Failure to complete skill assessment within ten minutes.

Evaluator's Signature: Date:

Spinal Motion Restriction: Supine

Name: Date: Start Time: End Time: Evaluator's Name:

Critical Failure Criteria in Bold	If Completed	Points Missed
1. Demonstrates body substance isolation precautions		AF
2. Directs assistant to maintain manual cervical spine immobilization		AF
3. Assesses patient's circulation, sensory, and motor function: a. Circulation: presence of distal pulses in each extremity b. Sensory: patient feels physical stimuli applied to fingers and toes c. Motor: patient able move hands and feet		AF

4. Applies appropriate size cervical collar
   a. Measures first
   b. Applies from the front of the patient's neck		

5. Place's backboard beside patient with top of board located approximately 3 inches above top of patient's head		

6. Log rolls patient onto side toward rescuers
   a. Directs assistant at body to support hips and legs
   b. Directs assistant at head to coordinate log roll
   c. Controls patient's torso and hips		

7. Inspects/palpates/auscultates patient's back for injury/bleeding/breath sounds		
8. Instructs assistant at head to direct log roll onto backboard		
9. Secures body to backboard using appropriate straps		
10. Pads all voids		
11. Immobilizes head and neck to backboard using appropriate appliance		
12. Instructs assistant at head to release manual stabilization		

13. Reassesses patient's circulation, sensory, and motor function		AF
Total Points		100

Critical Fail Criteria

- Failure to manage the patient as a competent EMT.
- Exhibits unacceptable affect with patient or other personnel.
- Uses or orders a dangerous or inappropriate intervention.
- Failure to immobilize head and neck to backboard.
- Failure to complete skill assessment within ten minutes.

Evaluator's Signature: Date:

Spinal Motion Restriction: Seated/KED

Name: Date: Start Time: End Time: Evaluator's Name:

Critical Failure Criteria in Bold	If Completed	Points Missed
1. Demonstrates body substance isolation precautions		AF
2. Directs assistant to maintain manual cervical spine immobilization		AF
3. Assesses patient's circulation, sensory, and motor function: a. Circulation: presence of distal pulses in each extremity		AF

b. Sensory: patient feels physical stimuli applied to fingers and toes c. Motor: patient able move hands and feet		

4. Applies appropriate size cervical collar
    a. Measures first
    b. Applies from the front of the patient's neck		

5. Places immobilization device behind patient, with "wings" of vest placed directly under patient axillae		
6. Applies middle torso strap		
7. Applies bottom torso strap		
8. Applies leg straps		
9. Immobilizes head and neck to vest, filling voids between head and vest first		
10. Instructs patient to take a deep breath		
11. Applies top torso strap		
12. Directs assistant to release manual stabilization		
13. Reassesses patient's circulation, sensory, and motor function		AF

If appropriate to move patient to backboard per spinal motion restriction protocol, follow steps 12-15

14. Moves patient to supine position on backboard, supports legs while positioning patient		
15. Releases leg straps		
16. Secures patient to backboard		
17. Reassesses patient's circulation, sensory, and motor function		AF
Total Points		100

Critical Fail Criteria

- Failure to manage the patient as a competent EMT.
- Exhibits unacceptable affect with patient or other personnel.
- Uses or orders a dangerous or inappropriate intervention.
- Failure to complete skill assessment within ten minutes.

Evaluator's Signature: Date:

Traction Splint

Name: Date: Start Time: End Time: Evaluator's Name:

Critical Failure Criteria in Bold	If Completed	Points Missed
1. Demonstrates body substance isolation precautions		AF
Examiner asks for indications for use of traction splint		
2. Verbalizes indications for use of traction splint a. Femur fracture that is		AF

	b. Isolated c. Closed d. Mid-shaft	
3.	Directs application of manual stabilization *(no manual traction)*	AF

4.	Assesses patient circulatory, sensory, and motor function prior to application of traction splint
	   a. Circulation: presence of distal pulses in each extremity
	   b. Sensory: patient feels physical stimuli applied to fingers and toes
	   c. Motor: patient able move hands and feet
		AF

The examiner states, "Circulatory, sensory, and motor function are present."		
5.	Prepares/adjusts splint to the proper length measured to non-injured leg	
6.	Positions the splint underneath the injured leg	
7.	Applies the proximal securing device/ischial strap properly	
8.	Applies the distal securing device/ankle hitch properly	
9.	Applies mechanical traction appropriately	

10. Positions/secures the support straps		
11. Re-evaluates the proximal/distal securing devices		
12. Reassesses circulatory, sensory, and motor function in the injured leg		AF
The examiner states "Circulatory, sensory, and motor function are present." *The examiner must ask the candidate how he/she would prepare the patient for transportation*		
13. Verbalizes securing the torso to the long board to immobilize the hip		
14. Verbalizes securing the splint to the long board to prevent movement of Th e splint		
Total Points		100

Critical Fail Criteria:

- Failure to manage the patient as a competent EMT.
- Exhibits unacceptable affect with patient or other personnel.
- Uses or orders a dangerous or inappropriate intervention.
- Failure to complete skill assessment within ten minutes.
- Inability to achieve traction.
- Positions strap over injury site.
- Positions strap over joint.
- Excessive movement/manipulation.

Evaluator's Signature: Date:

Obstetrical Emergencies: Childbirth

Name: Date: Start Time: End Time: Evaluator's Name:

Critical Failure Criteria in Bold	If Completed	Points Missed
1. Demonstrates body substance isolation precautions		AF

2. Determines if delivery is imminent
   a. Crowning
   b. Urge to bear down or move bowels
   c. Bloody show
   d. Severe low back pain
		AF

3. Verbalizes, if applicable, any presentation other than head, along with appropriate concerns & interventions (Prolapsed cord, breech, etc.)		

4. Identifies the following:
   a. Pre-natal care/expected complications
   b. Due date
   c. Gravida and para (number of pregnancies, number of live births)		

5. If hypoxic, provide oxygen for mother as indicated		
6. Place mother in position of comfort. Prepare area/equipment for delivery (Blanket/chux, OB kit from ambulance)		

7.	Supports baby's head, applies gentle pressure to perineum to prevent tearing, verbalizes position of cord and properly corrects if necessary		
8.	Assists in delivery of shoulders and torso		
9.	Dry and cover newborn for warmth (especially the head). If possible, place skin-to-skin with the mother on abdomen or to breast for shared body heat. Wrap mother and baby together.		
10.	Assess baby's one minute APGAR score (Appearance, Pulse, Grimace, Activity, Respiration). Verbalizes any immediate intervention as appropriate		AF
11.	Allow cord to pulse for at least 1 minute OR until pulsing stops. To cut cord, clamp cord with 2 clamps, cut between both clamps, approximately 6-8 inches from baby (If cord interferes with neonatal resuscitation, cut immediately)		
12.	Assesses mother's vital signs		
13.	Determines appropriate transport code and hospital destination		
14.	Assess baby's five minute APGAR score		AF

15. Allows for spontaneous delivery of placenta, bags, and brings with patients to hospital (Do not delay transport to hospital for delivery of placenta)		
16. If bleeding persists post-delivery of placenta, rub abdomen below navel w i t h flat hand x15 seconds as needed		
17. Reassess mother and baby		
Total Points		100

Critical Fail Criteria

- Failure to manage the patient as a competent EMT.
- Exhibits unacceptable affect with patient or other personnel.
- Uses or orders a dangerous or inappropriate intervention.
- Failure to complete skill assessment within ten minutes.

Evaluator's Signature: Date:

Needle Cricothyrotomy with Jet Insufflation

Name: Date: Start Time: End Time: Evaluator's Name:

Critical Failure Criteria in Bold	If Completed	Points Missed
1. Demonstrates body substance isolation precautions		AF

2.	Verbalizes indications: Severe airway obstruction where all BLS and ALS attempts to secure airway were unsuccessful.		
3.	Connects modified regulator to oxygen cylinder		
4.	Connect jet insufflator to discharge outlet on modified regulator		
5.	Connect extension tubing with stopcock to jet insufflator		
6.	Adjust pressure gauge to appropriate psi (50 psi for adults vs. 20 psi for children). A child is 14 year or younger in SF Protocols		AF
7.	Have the stopcock set in the appropriate direction for initial ventilation to the patient's lungs		
8.	Attach the appropriate size cricothyroidotomy needle (adult vs. child size) to the 10cc syringe. While keeping needle sterile, hands it to the paramedic		
9.	Locate and clean the cricothyroid membrane area with alcohol preps		
Paramedic performs needle cricothyrotomy			
10.	Open the oxygen tank		

Paramedic presses the jet button, inflates until minimal chest rise observed		
11. Following the ventilation, assists the paramedic by rotating stopcock to allow for five second exhalation (or briefly disconnect if no stopcock)		
12. Assists by gently pressing down on the patient's chest to allow for depressurization as necessary		
13. Rotate stopcock for ventilation		
14. Repeat jet insufflation techniques until the resuscitation has been terminated or until airway has been transferred to a higher level of care.		
Total Points		100

Critical Fail Criteria

- Failure to manage the patient as a competent EMT.
- Exhibits unacceptable affect with patient or other personnel.
- Uses or orders a dangerous or inappropriate intervention.
- Failure to complete skill assessment within ten minutes.

Evaluator's Signature: Date:

Chapter 34

POST-TRAUMATIC STRESS DISORDER

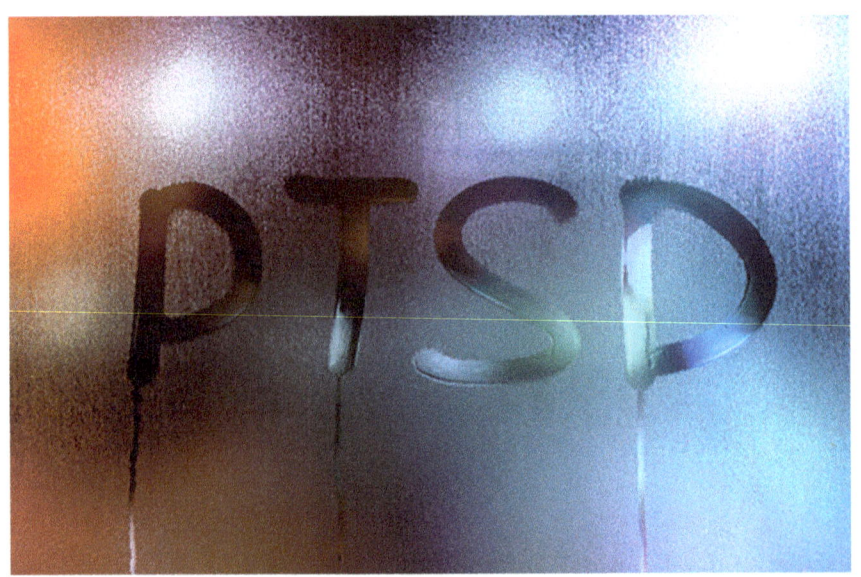

254 | MARK POYER

Here it is. The one thing that no one ever talks about. It's taboo. It's weakness. How dare we feel human. If we feel we cannot perform our job, right? Let's get real for a second. PTSD in first responders is very real. PTSD can affect anyone. So if you start to notice signs and symptoms, don't wait to get help (see resources below). It does not matter if it's your first day or if you're thirty years in. Everyone's trauma can be different. Everyone has different triggers. But please understand that this is a real risk getting into this line of work. It does not matter if you're a firefighter, EMT, paramedic, police officer, veteran, or a dispatcher. *The only person who will take care of yourself is you.* If you struggle in your career, please reach out, don't isolate yourself. With that out of the way, let's begin.

Now I don't know about you, but when I was in school, the amount of time we spent on the subject of PTSD was pretty much nonexistent. I mean, come on. It was way more important to know those drug calculations or where to locate those damn fallopian tubes on the ambulance (EMS joke). In all seriousness, I do not even remember covering the subject. You see, being in school is very different from working on the streets. We are there on people's worst days, but you know that when you start school right? Let's talk about what you may not be prepared for.

School does not prepare you to see or smell dead decomposing bodies. School does not prepare you to tell a new mother that her baby girl just died after they spent the last ten years trying to have children. School does not prepare you to walk in on a child who shot himself in the head playing with dad's firearm. School does not prepare you for the number of times you will get assaulted by patients who you are trying to help. School does not prepare you to tell a wife and her children that their dad died swimming in the ocean immediately after doing CPR for over an hour and a half. Have you ever pulled an eight-month-old out of a boiling pot of water in the kitchen because the psychotic mother said her kid wouldn't stop crying so she was punishing him? I have. These stories can go on and on. You see the trend here. But most importantly, school does not prepare you for how to properly handle these things at the end of the day when you go home.

So let me ask you this, What do you do on these calls? You do your job, right? You put your emotions aside because we need to focus on our job—on being professional. We are always in the public's eye. There is no time to be weak. You see, here's the double-edged sword. We become extremely good at setting our emotions to the side, pushing them down. We joke about terrible things as a way to cope. That sick sense of humor. You know how it is.

But you know, these calls bug you, or maybe not everyone is different. Maybe these thoughts are always in the back of your mind. Maybe they pop up from time to time, maybe they prevent you from going places, or wanting to leave your home. Maybe they make you want to isolate or be away from your friends or family. Maybe you just feel tired and lethargic all the time? Must be normal because of all the long hours we work, right? Not enough caffeine in the world to keep you alert. Let us talk about sleep. What is sleep anyway? Hey, if you find out, let me know. In all seriousness, very poor sleep. Easily woken up even to the smallest noises. Nightmares? Yeah, we get the best ones.

It can be exhausting. Twelve- to twenty-four-hour long shifts multiple days per week, mandatory overtime regularly. Burnout. High stress environment. Maybe it is causing issues at home. Maybe you drink to drown the thoughts out? Maybe you start using drugs? Maybe you're super aggressive and irritable all the time? Maybe you're consumed by rage. Everything pisses you off. Do you ever get angry when a call gets dispatched? Is that normal for you? Maybe you start a pattern of calling out sick, or maybe you pick up more shifts? I mean, when you are constantly working, there is no time to stop and deal with the thoughts, right? Maybe the thoughts play in your head repeatedly like you are constantly rewatching a terrible movie on repeat all day from the second you wake up till you go to bed to the point where you just want it to stop. Maybe you become numb to everything—no longer showing emotion. Maybe your current coping mechanisms stop working for you, and now you're just drowning in your thoughts. You feel empty, or maybe you have become so depressed that nothing is important anymore. Not your significant other, not your kids, not your family, not your friends, not your dog, not yourself. Maybe you become suicidal. Now there is a serious topic.

Oh, man, have I been there. Funny thing is I didn't even think I had PTSD. When I found out I actually had PTSD, I was in disbelief. I told myself, *Nah that's just for veterans who are like twenty-five to thirty years in*. My wife would say otherwise after watching me jump out of a moving vehicle at 25 mph to confront someone who cut my wife off while driving. Yeah, you heard that right. I did it. My wife wouldn't pull over so I could go yell at the guy, so I jumped out. I was stupid and reckless. But you know what, he deserved it! Totally kidding. Unfortunately, when PTSD gets severe, a part of your brain shuts off. The logical reasoning part, the amygdala and the prefrontal cortex. And all you see is red, and you act before you even have a second to think. That was my wake-up moment. Am I embarrassed by it? Definitely. Will I do it again? Nope. Because I reached out when I needed to. I share this embarrassing story with you because I don't want you to get to the point of having a wake-up moment because I could have died jumping out of the car, and the road rash was no joke, and I looked like an idiot.

Now before I dive into PTSD a bit more, I want you to understand that there are multiple types of PTSD which I will list below. There is a normal stress response, acute stress disorder, uncomplicated PTSD, complex PTSD, and comorbid PTSD. I deal with complex PTSD. Multiple calls and situations over an eleven-year career working with many different agencies in different areas over my career. You see, sometimes it just creeps up on you, and you are not even aware of it. And sometimes a single call can be your trigger. It doesn't need to be many.

Having a PTSD diagnosis is like being on a roller coaster sometimes. You see, I'm a perfectionist. I'd like to say a lot of us in the medical field are because we need to be. We don't get to make mistakes. When we make mistakes, people get hurt or have bad outcomes. There's another double-edged sword. A lot of my ups and downs involved me getting frustrated and pissed off at myself when I'm not getting better fast enough. I was trying to feel like the old me (pre-PTSD), which isn't possible by the way, but this is the reality. It can consume you day in and day out, and once you have it, it's yours to keep. The repetitive thoughts, the fears, the anxiety, the depression, it lingers.

But here is the good news. You don't need to strive to become the old version of yourself. Focus on being the new and improved you. Throughout my healing process, I have been working on becoming a better person, a better father, and a better husband. I have become better. You adapt, and you learn to take care of you. And even though the symptoms are there, they can be managed in a healthy way. If you have triggers, learn what they are. Learn how to manage them. Go outside, spend time with friends and family, laugh, workout, take vacations when you need them, be spontaneous, and enjoy life to the fullest. The job will always be there when you get back. Focus on yourself and know that there are plenty of resources available for us to utilize if we need them. Once again, I am not trying to deter you from this career choice. For every really bad call, I have hundreds of amazing calls. I have met some of the most amazing people on this planet in this line of work. This job is exciting, and there is nothing else like it.

Now understand I am not trying to scare you. I am sharing my experiences with you so if you ever notice these things and start to struggle, you know that you are not alone. There are thousands just like you, just like me. You are not different or weak for having these issues arise. Recognize signs and symptoms. Find healthy coping mechanisms. Focus on you and your health. If you need help, get it. This job is one of the best jobs in the world—a true calling—but it does have risks, and this is one of them. Understand that this job is not for everyone, and it is okay to walk away. It's okay to take a break if you need it. It is okay to feel emotions and feel human. But at the end of the day, if you want to have a long healthy career, you need to be strong both physically and mentally.

Post-Traumatic Stress Disorder (PTSD)

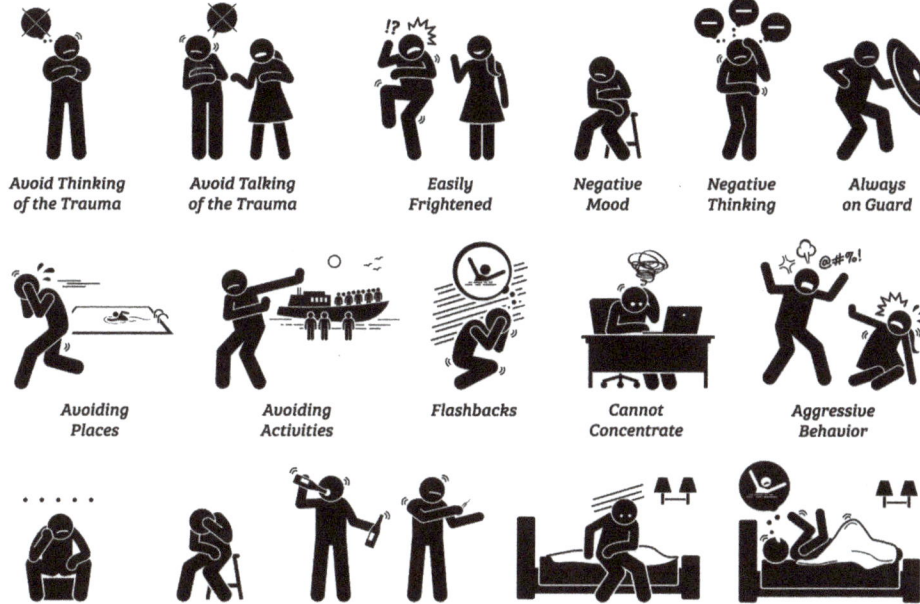

PTSD Signs and Symptoms

1	Intrusive thoughts
2	Detachment of others/disassociation (disconnecting from thoughts, feelings, memories, or sense of identity)
3	Irritability, rage, angry outbursts, and feeling on edge
4	Hypervigilance
5	Anxiety
6	Insomnia, restlessness, and trouble falling asleep or staying asleep
7	Feeling numb, distant, and cutting off from others

8	Depression, hopelessness, and feelings of guilt or shame
9	No longer enjoy activities you used to enjoy
10	Suicidal ideation
11	Poor memory, difficulty concentrating, and losing things often
12	Easily startled, agitated, and jumpy
13	Feeling on guard
14	Experiencing rapid heartbeat, tight breathing, and upset stomach
15	Loss of appetite
16	Substance abuse
17	Reoccurring memories of traumatic events
18	Flashbacks
19	Bad dreams or nightmares
20	Easily triggered by things that remind you of the trauma

Brain Regions Affected by PTSD

Amygdala is a small, almond-shaped region of the brain that plays a role in several functions, including:	• Some mating functions • The assessment of threat-related stimuli (i.e., assessing what in the environment is considered a danger) • The formation and storage of emotional memories • Fear conditioning • Memory consolidation

Prefrontal Cortex (PFC) is an area of the brain found in the frontal lobe. This region of the brain plays an important part in PTSD. Some of the key functions of the prefrontal cortex include:	• Emotional regulation • Initiating voluntary, conscious behaviors • Regulating attention • Decision-making • Interpreting emotions
Hippocampus is complex brain structure embedded deep into the temporal lobe. It has a major role in learning and memory. It is a plastic and vulnerable structure that gets damaged by a variety of stimuli.	The hippocampus helps regulate smell, spatial coding, and memory. More specifically, the hippocampus helps store long-term memories, basically helping to decide what goes from being a short-term memory to what becomes a long-term memory. This process of turning short-term memory into long-term memory is what is referred to as memory consolidation. Damage to the hippocampus can also release excess cortisol (a stress hormone).

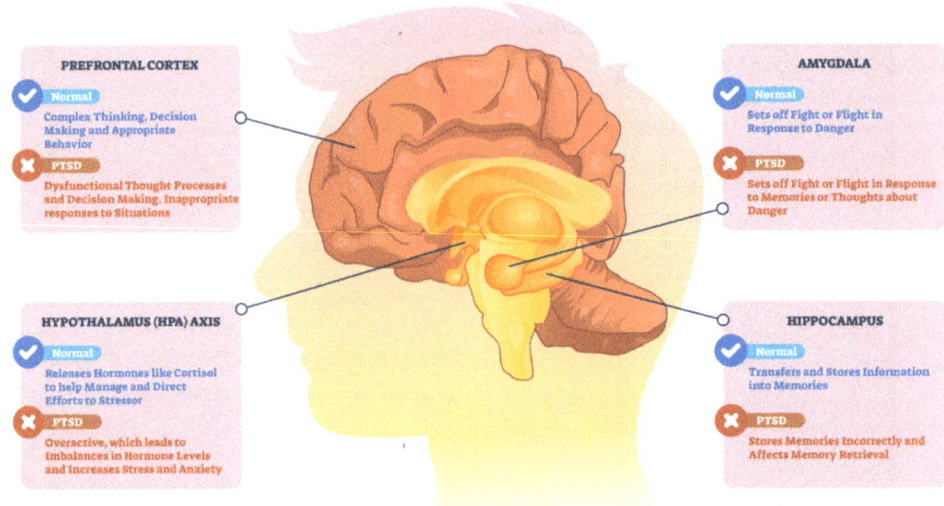

PTSD
Posttraumatic Stress Disorder

Posttraumatic Stress Disorder (PTSD) is a Mental Disorder that can Develop After a Person is Exposed to a Traumatic Event

PREFRONTAL CORTEX
- Normal: Complex Thinking, Decision Making and Appropriate Behavior
- PTSD: Dysfunctional Thought Processes and Decision Making, Inappropriate responses to Situations

AMYGDALA
- Normal: Sets off Fight or Flight in Response to Danger
- PTSD: Sets off Fight or Flight in Response to Memories or Thoughts about Danger

HYPOTHALAMUS (HPA) AXIS
- Normal: Releases Hormones like Cortisol to help Manage and Direct Efforts to Stressor
- PTSD: Overactive, which leads to Imbalances in Hormone Levels and Increases Stress and Anxiety

HIPPOCAMPUS
- Normal: Transfers and Stores Information into Memories
- PTSD: Stores Memories Incorrectly and Affects Memory Retrieval

Potential Causes of PTSD

 War

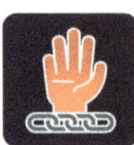 Sexual Abuse

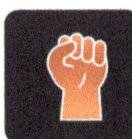 Physical Abuse

 Emotional Abuse

 Robbery or Burglary

 Witnessing or Experiencing Mass Disasters

 Separation

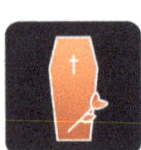 Death of a Loved One

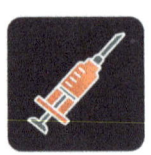 Medical Procedure

 Witnessing or Experiencing A Serious Accident

Types of PTSD

Normal stress response	Occurs before PTSD begins. It does not always lead up to the full disorder. Events like accidents, injuries, illnesses, surgeries, and other sources of unreasonable amounts of tension and stress can all lead to this response. A normal stress response can be effectively managed with the support of loved ones, peers, and individual or group therapy sessions. Individuals suffering from normal stress response should see a recovery within a few weeks.
Acute stress disorder	Not the same as PTSD. It can occur in people who have been exposed to what is or what feels like a life-threatening event. Natural disasters, loss of loved ones, loss of a job, or risk of death are all stressors that can trigger acute stress disorder. If left untreated, acute stress disorder may develop into PTSD. Acute stress disorder can be treated through individual and group therapy, medication, and intensive treatments designed by a psychiatrist.
Uncomplicated PTSD	Uncomplicated PTSD is linked to one major traumatic event versus multiple events and is the easiest form of PTSD to treat. Symptoms of uncomplicated PTSD include avoidance of trauma reminders, nightmares, flashbacks to the event, irritability, mood changes, and changes in relationships. Uncomplicated PTSD can be treated through therapy, medication, or a combination of both.

Complex PTSD	Complex PTSD is the opposite of uncomplicated PTSD. It is caused by multiple traumatic events, not just one. Complex PTSD is common in abuse or domestic violence cases, repeated exposure to war or community violence, or sudden loss. While they share the same symptoms, treatment of complex PTSD is a little more intense than uncomplicated PTSD. Individuals with complex PTSD can be diagnosed with borderline or antisocial personality disorder or dissociative disorders. They exhibit behavioral issues such as impulsivity, aggression, substance abuse, or sexual impulsivity. They can also exhibit extreme emotional issues such as intense rage, depression, or panic.
Comorbid PTSD	Comorbid PTSD is a blanket term for co-occurring disorders. It is applied when a person has more than one mental health concern, often coupled with substance abuse issues. Comorbid PTSD is extremely common as many people suffer from more than one condition at a time. Best results are achieved when both the commingling mental health condition and the comorbid PTSD are treated at the same time. Many people who suffer from PTSD try to treat it on their own. This can include self-medication and other destructive behaviors. Using drugs or alcohol as a way to numb the pain will only make things worse and prolong treatment.

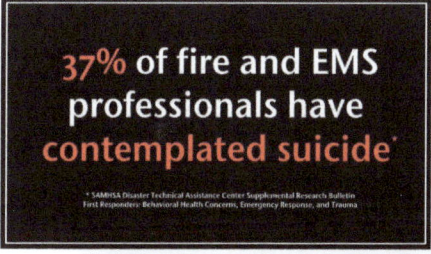
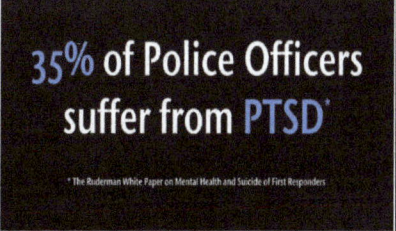
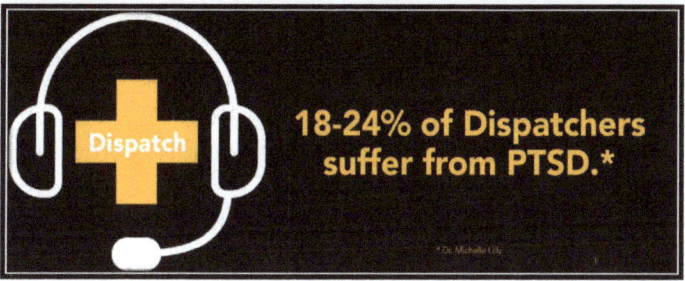

Coping Strategies

Meditation	A practice where an individual uses a technique such as mindfulness or focusing the mind on a particular object, thought, or activity to train attention and awareness and achieve a mentally clear and emotionally calm and stable state.
Tactical breathing	A method that focuses on slowing the breathing rate down by inhaling through the nostrils for four seconds and exhaling out the mouth for four seconds. Use during stressful situations. This stimulates the vagus nerve and reduces anxiety and increases the parasympathetic system.

Grounding exercises	There are many grounding exercises. When you start to have a panic attack, stop and focus on tactical breathing. Close your eyes. Just listen to your surroundings. Think about what you are hearing. Think about what you're smelling. Open your eyes, look around the room. What do you see? Table, chair, couch? Repeat those steps. Shift your focus. Find your peace.
5-4-3-2-1 method	Working backward from five, use your senses to list things you notice around you. For example, you might start by listing five things you hear, then four things you see, then three things you can touch from where you're sitting, two things you can smell, and one thing you can taste. Make an effort to notice the little things you might not always pay attention to such as the color of the flecks in the carpet or the hum of your computer.
Laugh	Enables us to experience joy, and joy feels like a glimmer of hope to the individual who is trapped within the anxious paralysis of PTSD. Find a funny video to watch. Look up some jokes.
Music	Can reduce symptoms and improve **functioning among individuals with trauma exposure and** PTSD. Music can reduce depression symptoms and improving health-related quality of life.

Exercise	Regular exercise can also have a positive impact on your mental health by reducing anxiety and depression. In one study of adults with PTSD, a twelve-week exercise program that included three thirty-minute resistance training sessions a week, as well as walking, was found to lead to a significant decrease in PTSD symptoms, depression, and better sleep quality after the program ended.
Support groups	You are not alone. There are tons of first responder support groups available. It is tremendously helpful to know there are others out there dealing with the same issues. Don't isolate. Reach out to your peers.
Writing	Using journaling to cope with and express your thoughts and feelings (also called expressive writing) can be a good way of coping with PTSD. Expressive writing has been found to improve physical and psychological health. In PTSD in particular, expressive writing has been found to have a number of benefits, including improved coping, post-traumatic growth (the ability to find meaning in and have positive life changes following a traumatic event), and reduced PTSD symptoms, tension, and anger.

1-degree of change	I want you to stop and think about a compass. If you veer off 1-degree for a long enough period, you will land in a much different spot. When you are approaching treatment, sometimes the things you have been doing aren't working anymore. Veer off on that 1-degree change. For example, say you feel like isolating because you're having repetitive thoughts and want to be alone. Instead reach out to someone, talk to your spouse, go hang out with a friend. Do something different. Overtime you will change and get better.

PTSD Treatment

EMDR therapy (eye movement desensitization and reprocessing)	Psychotherapy that enables people to heal from the symptoms and emotional distress that are the result of disturbing life experiences. Repeated studies show that by using EMDR therapy people can experience the benefits of psychotherapy that once took years to make a difference. EMDR has a very high success rate for treatment. It allows your brain to reprocess the trauma and helps you begin to heal and maybe even have a completely different outlook on the traumatic event. Highly recommend this treatment method.
Medications	Let's be honest here, our brains are wired differently. We process threats differently, our body's chemicals are out of balance, and our fight our flight response is triggered way faster. Medication can help with depression, anxiety, nightmares, and flashbacks. They can help you get better sleep. They can help you have a more positive outlook on life. Understand that medication

	is like a Band-Aid. Medication can help you get to a position to where you can focus on your own healing process. You do not need to stay on it permanently.
Cognitive behavioral therapy	The idea is to change the thought patterns that are disturbing your life. This might happen through talking about your trauma or concentrating on where your fears come from. The goals are to: • Improve your symptoms, • Teach you skills to deal with it, and • Restore your self-esteem.
Cognitive processing therapy	CPT is a twelve-week course of treatment with weekly sessions of sixty to ninety minutes. You'll talk about the traumatic event with your therapist and how your thoughts related to it have affected your life. Then you'll write in detail about what happened. This process helps you examine how you think about your trauma and figure out new ways to live with it. It helps you understand that things were beyond your control, so you can move forward; understanding and accepting that, deep down, it wasn't your fault despite things you did or didn't do.
Prolonged exposure therapy	If you've been avoiding things that remind you of the traumatic event, then this treatment is for you. It involves eight to fifteen sessions, usually ninety minutes each. Your therapist will teach you techniques to ease your anxiety and your symptoms, and you will dive deep into the trauma and how it's affected your life, and you will learn how to face it.

PTSD Resources

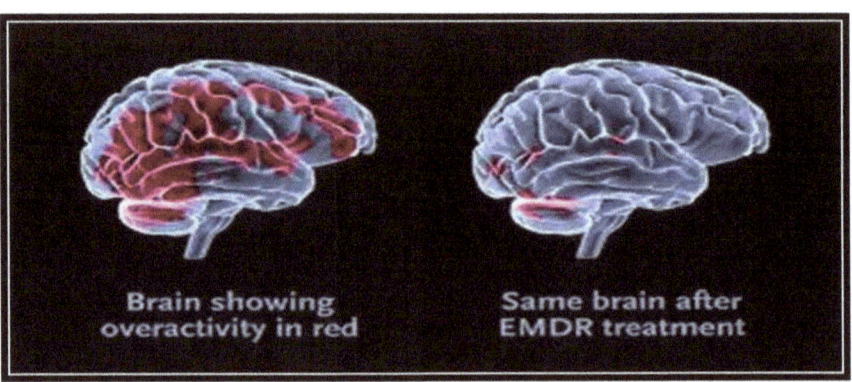

Brain showing overactivity in red — Same brain after EMDR treatment

WCPR (The West Coast Post-Trauma Retreat)	The WCPR program is for first responders whose lives have been affected by their work experience. The WCPR residential program provides an educational experience designed to help current and retired first responders recognize the signs and symptoms of work-related stress including post-traumatic stress disorder (PTSD) in themselves and in others. There are many locations throughout the United States and is one of the best resources you can take advantage of if you struggle with PTSD.
Books	• *CopShock, Second Edition: Surviving Post-Traumatic Stress Disorder (PTSD)* • *Emotional Survival for Law Enforcement: A Guide for Officers and Their Families* • *I Love a Fire Fighter: What the Family Needs to Know* • *I Love a Cop, Revised Edition: What Police Families Need to Know* • *Surviving the Shadows: A Journey of Hope into Post-Traumatic Stress*

	- *The Body Keeps the Score* by Bessel Van Der Kolk (healing from trauma)
- *The Dance of Anger* by Harriet Lerner (anger issues)
- *The Tapping Solution* by Nick Ortner (grounding change from negative to positive)
- *Forgive for Good* by Frederic Luskin (forgiveness)
- *Outgrowing the Pain* by Eliana Gil (child abuse)
- *Embracing Your Inner Critic* by Hal Stone (self-criticism)
- *The 5 Languages of Love* by Gary Chapman (relationships and communication)
- *The 7 Principles for Making Marriage Work* by John Gottman (relationships)
Addiction centers	- http://www.addictioncenter.com/, (877) 544-0037
- https://mountainvistafarm.com/
- Alcohol and Drug Recovery Center located in Sonoma, (800) 300-6716
- https://www.serenityknolls.com/
- California's Best 12-Step Drug And Alcohol Treatment Center located in Marin, (855) 552-7901
EMDR Institute	Website: https://www.emdr.com/ Founded by Dr. Francine Shapiro in 1990, offers quality trainings in the EMDR therapy methodology, a treatment approach that has been empirically validated in over thirty randomized studies of trauma victims. You can find tons of information regarding EMDR here.

The Overwatch Collective (A podcast made for First Responders)	*The Overwatch Collective started out as a podcast hosted by two active members of the military. Greg and Jesse set out to help individuals across all areas of public service from Military, Fire, EMT, Paramedics, Law Enforcement, Corrections Officers, and Dispatchers, as well as the spouses and family members of the people who serve so selflessly. We simply started sharing stories, experiences, and resources, and our podcast soon grew into a family.* *Our motto is "One more is one less" because if we can help just one person feel a little less alone, it could end up saving their life.*
Badge of Life	Website: https://badgeoflife.org/ Our mission is to educate and train law enforcement about mental health and suicide prevention. No more broken cops or cops' families. Lots of resources available for police officers.
Code 9	Website: https://code9.org/ Making first responder mental health a priority. Our mission is to work toward positive change in the first responder culture as we continue to raise awareness, advocate, and educate on the devastating effects of PTSD for first responders and families that could lead to suicide. We are working with many others toward making real change a reality.
COPS	Website: https://www.concernsofpolicesurvivors.org/ Rebuilding shattered lives (lots of available Material for law enforcement officers both retired and currently working).

PISTLE	Post-Incident Stress and Trauma in Law Enforcement Website: https://www.pistle.org/ PISTLE-PS is a nonprofit organization dedicated to providing resources for law enforcement and public safety professionals who are battling the effects of stress from critical incidents incurred in the line of duty. The staff at PISTLE-PS are current or retired law enforcement officers and firefighters who have experienced and understand the stress involved from enduring critical incidents.
Responder Strong	Website: https://you.responderstrong.org/ Prioritize your well-being with personalized tips, tools, and advice from other responders and healthcare workers, 100 percent free and confidential.
Numbers to Call	• Safe Call Now: 1-206-459-3020. A 24-7 helpline staffed by first responders for first responders and their family members. They can assist with treatment options for responders who are suffering from mental health, substance abuse, and other personal issues. • Fire/EMS helpline: 1-888-731-3473. Also known as Share the Load, a program run by the National Volunteer Fire Council. They have a helpline, text-based help service, and also collected a list of many good resources for people looking for help and support.

- National Suicide Prevention Lifeline: 1-800-273-8255. The national (USA) suicide hotline. Not first responder specific, but they can and will talk to anyone who needs help. We've been told by one of their founders they have a large number of first responders and veterans who volunteer.
- Crisis text line service that allows people in crisis to speak with a trained crisis counselor by texting "Start" or "Help" to 741-741.
- Copline (law enforcement only): **1-800-267-5463**. A confidential helpline for members of US law enforcement. Their website also has additional information on help and resources.
- Frontline Helpline: 1-866-676-7500. Run by Frontline Responder Services. Offers 24-7 coverage with first responder call takers.
- Kristin Brooks Hopeline: 1-800-442-4673. Another national (USA) hotline for people suffering from mental health issues.
- Veterans Crisis Line (veterans only): 1-800-273-8255 and press 1 or text 838255. A crisis line specifically for veterans of the US armed forces.

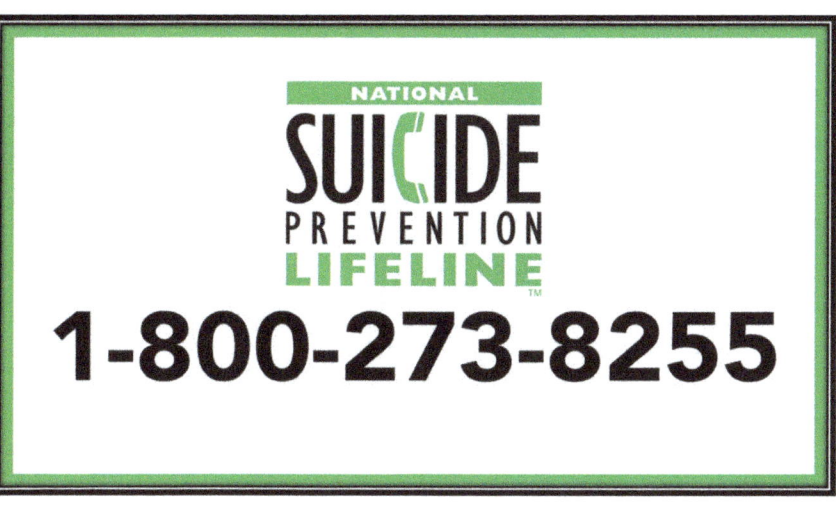

Do not be afraid to reach out for help. Your life matters.

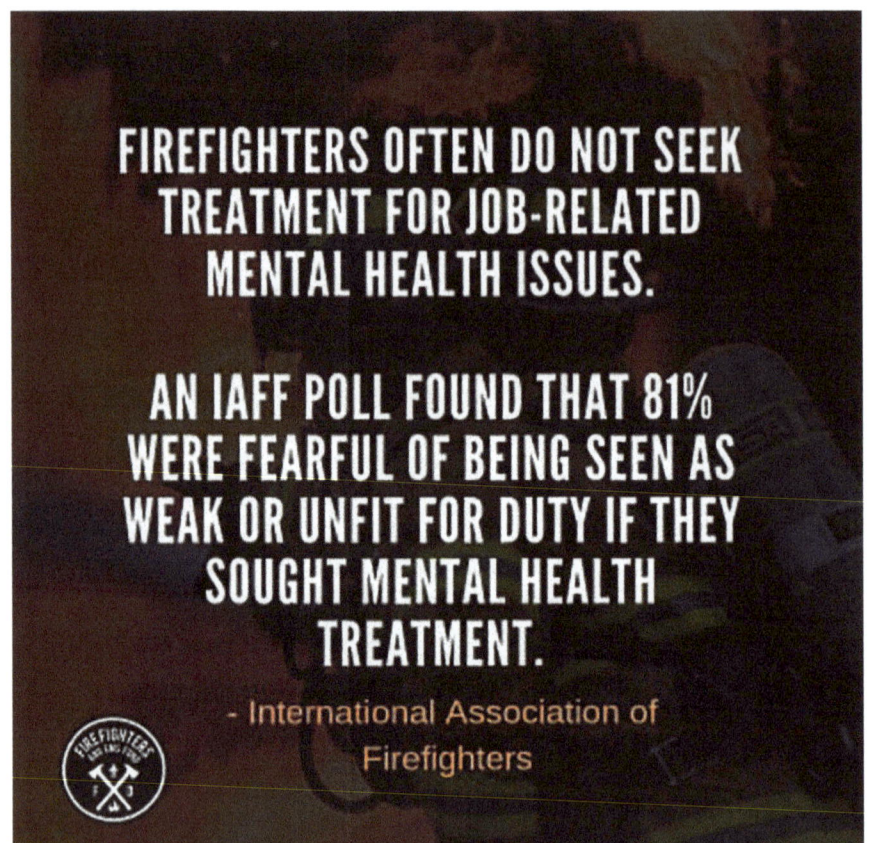

About the Author

My name is Mark Poyer. I am married with four beautiful daughters. I grew up in the Bay Area and have been involved in fire and emergency medical services for the last ten years. I have ambulance experience as an EMT and a paramedic working both BLS and ALS working with Rural Metro, AMR, and Paramedics Plus. I completed my internship at Paramedics Plus. I have since worked in several different counties including Alameda County, Contra Costa County, Solano County, Santa Clara County, and the city and county of San Francisco. I have also worked with multiple fire departments in many different positions from being with Cal Fire to being a firefighter and engineer as a volunteer with the River Delta Fire District. I currently work for the San Francisco Fire Department and have been a paramedic, FTO, and preceptor there for over five years now. It is extremely important to me to give back to the community as well as to help other individuals become successful in our line of work, which is why this book was created. It is a tool that I wish I had upon embarking on my internship and is a product that I know many students carry with them today.

www.ingramcontent.com/pod-product-compliance
Lightning Source LLC
Chambersburg PA
CBHW040107180526
45172CB00009B/1255